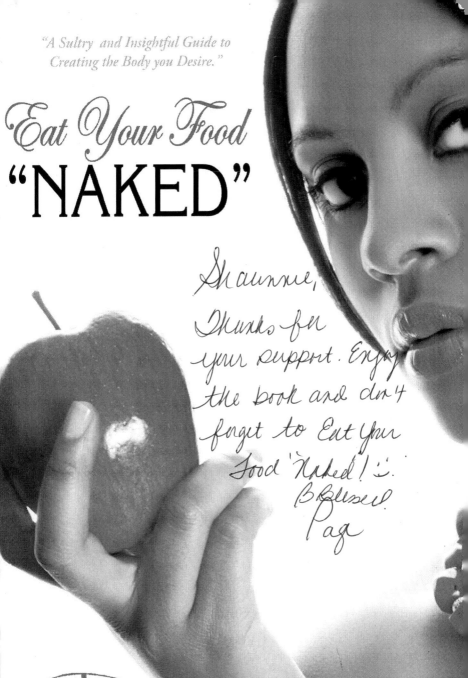

*"A Sultry and Insightful Guide to Creating the Body you Desire."*

# Eat Your Food
# "NAKED"

Shaunxie,
Thanks for
your support. Enjoy
the book and don't
forget to Eat Your
Food "Naked"! ☺.
B Blessed.
Page

## By
## Page

ISBN 13: 978-0-615-44767-4

Cover design: Marion Designs
Editor: Charmaine Parker
Author photos: Jeff Martin—Martin Photography
Cover model: S. Hasan—Facet Studio

Synergy Communications 1
11620 Reisterstown Road
Reisterstown, Maryland 21136
www.eatyourfoodnaked.com

# Gratitude

## My Mother
To my Mom, you are simply the best—thanks for giving me the world and exposing me to so many things at an early age. You made me the spoiled, determined, opinionated woman that I am! (smile) I will always love you.

## Stepfather
Noah Collins Jr., you are the only father I have ever known. You appeared in my mother's life and everything seemed easier. We miss you but Heaven must have needed an Angel.

## Sisters
Mya, thanks for being the inspiration behind my project. Karen (my special needs sister), you are the wind beneath my wings.

## Larry, Curly and Mo

My uncles John, Jesse and Roger, thank you for being the male figures in my life when no others were there. I don't know if that is a good or bad thing. Uncle Roger, you have spoiled me rotten and I love you for it. You are probably the reason why I am not married!

## Role Model

Joan Pratt, you are my Friend—My Sister—My Accountant—My Confidante—My Adviser—My Angel; you are what every woman should strive to be—such a Virtuous Woman… I LOVE YOU!

## Sister To Sister

Jamie Foster Brown, what can I say—my second mother, my sister, but most importantly, my friend, thank you for believing in me and giving me my first writing contract with *Sister2Sister Magazine*. You made so many things possible; you are a large part of my evolution.

## My Sparring Partner

Damon Moats, my friend and Partner for the past five years—thanks for getting in the ring with me and never throwing in the towel. You have listened to my ideas and supported me through this project—you will always be a very special part of my life.

## Chizel-It

Charles "Chizel-It" Harris, thanks for contributing to my project and keeping me in shape over the years. I would be a hot mess without you. :)
www.chizel-it.com

## My Author Girlfriends

Victoria Christopher Murray, thank you for helping me maximize my potential and start this journey. To my sister friend Zane, thank you for seeing me to the finish line—your talent is unprecedented. I WOULD HAVE NEVER FINISHED THIS WITHOUT YOU! You're simply the best! I truly admire you.

## Girlfriends

Karen Jefferson-Dina Jolley-Maisie Dunbar-Tania Collie-Renee Harris-Kim Pinkard-Melanie Few-Alice Bellamy-Malva Tuning-Sharon Green-Sarita Murray-Danita Williams-Sharon King-Dudley-Toi Crawford-Apryle Vaughn-Terri Sterling-Renault Daniels-Laquanda Murray-Stephanie Goldman-Robin Manzari-Lynn Smith-Bernadette Burrows-Cheloea Hill-Vickie Pouncie-Dr. Paula Orr
Where would I be without my Girlfriends!

## Brothers

To my Brothers from another mother—Attorney Warren Brown—Travis Winkey, thank you for helping build my foundation. Dr. Jamal Harrison Bryant—I consulted you on many projects. Thank you for consulting me on mine. Your resilience encourages me. Pastor Lloyd T. McGriff, thank you for being my spiritual brother. Stafford Sutton—smooth. Julius Henson, you *really* are a Teddy Bear with a heart of gold and I appreciate you.

## Cover Girl

My niece Maria Willis, thank you for being my Cover…Girl! You are Beautiful.
www.mariawillis.com

## Virtuous Woman

Nicola Jackson—your family values and Spiritual foundation are admired—thanks for pushing me in my Ardyss business. The Best is Yet to Come! … Sis

## My Ardyss Family

Let's continue to Create Wealth
While Promoting Health!

## Law & Order

Attorney Pam Fish, my sister and business partner, thank you for always being there and introducing me to Dr. LaJoyce Brookshire. Charmaine Parker, thank you for putting everything in order. If it were not for you, this book would still be pieces of paper on a kitchen table. You are the best in the business.

## Mentor

Terri Williams, thank you for showing me that a Black woman can make a gainful living without being an employee. You put Black Publicists on the map. Thanks for inspiring me early in my career.

## Project Managers

C. Hill and Chanay Robinson, thank you for putting up with my ADHD... sorry! We made it.

## My Donor

To my Father, thank you for not knowing me; in not knowing you, I grew to know Christ.
May you rest in Peace.

*You know God is all you need—when you look up and God is all you got!*
Unknown

"She's original, blunt, and funny as heck. A woman with strong determination and convictions dedicated to helping women beat the battle of the bulge! Page put the same power in this book that she puts in her workout. I love the question she asked: 'If your body was a piece of Real Estate—would you pass the Home Inspection?' Wow! If you're struggling with getting to the gym; *Eat Your Food Naked* is a must-read."

— Charles Harris
AFAA Certified Fitness Trainer

# Contents —

Welcome Aboard Naked Flight 36-24-36...............
Destination Weight Loss.

Please leave all Soft Drinks, Cookies, Cakes, Pies, and all negative baggage at the front of the cabin to be checked to your final destination by your Flight Attendants. Your flight is under the control of Captain Yoplait, assisted by First Officer Dannon. There are four Flight Attendants to assist you during the flight: Ben and Jerry and Baskin and Robbin. We have four emergency exits on board—two in the front of the cabin—fruits and vegetables, and two in the rear—sugars and carbohydrates. In case of extreme hunger, put your head in the bag in the seat pocket in front of you and count to ten. If there is any sign of overeating onboard, oxygen masks will be released from overhead. Please don your mask first, and then assist your child. In case of a water landing, the fat around your waist can be used as a flotation device. You may experience a bit of turbulence along the way, but don't let that deter you—just fasten your seatbelt—and enjoy the ride!

## Fasten Your Seatbelt

*E*at Your Food Naked! I knew that title would get your attention. Have you ever tried to eat your food naked? I know what you're thinking, but I don't mean for you to literally take off your clothes and warm up a plate. I used the sexy title to reel you in.

I see that it worked. Now that I have your attention, I need you to stick with me. I'll give you a full explanation behind the concept of the title later.

> How would **your weight differ** if you were penalized for every pound that you gained?

I wrote this book because, like millions of you, I am a sister who is trying to remain Fit, Fine, and Fabulous. Being over 40 and unmarried, I know that I have to keep it together for more than just health reasons. I never know when the time will come when I'll have to put this asset back on the market! I'm sure all of you single ladies know what I'm talking about, and some of you married ladies as well.

Let me ask you a question: How would your weight differ if you were penalized for every pound that you gained? You would be a lot thinner, wouldn't you? Well, that is somewhat the story of my life. You see, in my prior career, if I gained any substantial weight, there were monetary consequences to pay. If the weight gain became excessive, it could have cost me my job.

What career is that, you ask? Well, I had the good fortune of having that once most sought-after career—a Flight Attendant. Trust me; the job is not as glamorous as it seems. You know, I used to be one of those skinny, little girls strutting down the aisle asking, "Coffee, tea, or me?" Some of you may remember us better as stewardesses if you're part of the over-40 crowd.

You may not know this, but there was a time when, as a flight attendant, you were weighed annually. If you were found to be overweight, you were immediately put on suspension until your weight was back in line with the suggested weight scale. This meant that you were temporarily out of work until you "cut the fat." This may seem kind of harsh. It did to me, too, until I became mature enough to understand the importance of proper weight control.

I learned a lot from my co-workers, who were mostly Caucasian women. As an African-American woman, I grew up on fried chicken, macaroni and cheese, and biscuits and gravy— you know that good, old-fashioned, down-home soul food. So you can imagine my amazement as I watched my "clear" girlfriends make a meal out of carrots, celery, and peanut butter—literally! It seemed crazy to me then, but I learned many life lessons from my co-workers.

The examples that my co-workers set for me during my days as a Flight Attendant became part of my lifestyle and have helped me to control my weight into my 40s. I will not tell you how far into my 40s; that's none of your business. I am not saying that you can't ask; I'm saying that I might not answer. It's not that I am ashamed of my age; society puts limits and boundaries on you because of your age. And I refuse to be bound. Just know that I am almost one-half of 100—so you do the math! (smile)

I started flying when I was 21 years old, weighed 116 pounds, and wore a size 2. You may not believe this, but 20-plus years later, I am a size 4 and 125 pounds. Yes, God is good!

But I know what you're thinking: *She was always small,* or, *it's in her genes.*

You're right in one case: It is in my "jeans." It's in my size 4 jeans that I refuse to give up for a larger size. As far as my weight being hereditary, let me give you the family statistics, and then you can decide: My mother is about 5'6", weighs 240 pounds and wears a size 24 (sorry, Ma.) My oldest sister is about 5'6" and a size 16 on a good day. And my baby sister is 5'8", over 200 pounds and a size 20. She's really about a size 22, but she would kill me if I disclosed that top-secret information. So please keep this between us.

Let me say this before I forget: I am in no way saying I believe that everyone should be as skinny as a rail. I do, however, believe that everyone should be healthy! It is a known fact that weight gain has been linked to many preventable diseases, among them diabetes and high blood pressure. In many communities, these diseases are on the verge of becoming epidemic. Another thing that is historically true is that most people who live to be over 90 are not obese. I have never seen an octogenarian who weighed over 200 pounds! That should tell us something.

I am writing this book because, as a current Consultant for a Health and Wellness company, I deal with major obesity on a daily basis. It astounds me how little some people know about nutrition. I receive a lot of questions about my weight. It seems that nobody can believe my age because of my body composition. We have been programmed to believe that the older you are, the bigger you are supposed to be.

I believe that the larger you are, the older you look. You see, weight ages you. I believe that if you take off a few pounds, you will look and feel more youthful. Studies have shown that when you lose weight, you may gain confidence. That's not a bad exchange.

I think it's crazy when I hear women say that they are weighing their food, counting every calorie, going to meetings, getting B12 shots, etc.

All of this to lose weight? Who in the world has time? I mean, you don't want another job; you just want to lose weight... Right?

Maybe society has become so obese because the experts have made it too complicated to lose weight. It has become easier to be fat than to be fit. I think I have been able to help my friends, colleagues, and clients lose weight because my approach is very simple. You don't need a scale. You don't need a calorie counter. All you need is your Determination and a Desire to succeed.

I remember when I was a child my mother used to drag me every week to her Weight Watchers meetings. Her weight loss was very significant. So, I love Weight Watchers. I love Jenny Craig. They have great programs! But there is more than one way to skin a cat!

Before we go any further, let me say that I do realize that some weight gain is unavoidable. I do realize that women gain weight as they get older because of menopause and other factors dealt to us by nature. Certain medications are also known to increase weight gain. The birth of a child is also a major factor in weight retention in women. But, ladies, don't tell me you are overweight because you had a child and you have baby fat—and then I find out that your "baby" is about to graduate from college. That is sheer foolishness!

Let me say this: If you are a gym rat, this book may not be for you. This book is for the ladies, like me, who do not have time to pack a bag and run to the gym three times a week. I'm not saying that I never go to the gym. With my hectic schedule, I can't make it to the gym as much as I would like, but I am committed to staying in shape.

I used to go to the gym regularly, when I was between boyfriends and needed a date. I would put on my little workout gear, beat my face, and off I would go.

I was always successful. I would usually come out having not broken a sweat, but I would have a date for the weekend (smile). *You* know like *I* know that most gyms are pick-up spots—not all, but most. They are like meat markets, and unless you are a member of a gym that is unisex, nine times out of ten, working out is not the only thing on the members' minds.

A male friend of mine equates going to the gym to hanging out on South Beach. He said that

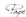

he goes to check out the body parts, and he *may* get a workout while he's there. (Boys are Dumb!)

I would love to share with you my secrets to weight maintenance. They have worked for me, and hopefully they will work for you. Like I said, I don't have time to go to the gym three times a week, but I do have time to find ways to stay in shape in the comfort of my own home. I don't live off of salad and fruit. I love food! I eat what I want. But there is a secret to that as well.

My accomplice, whom you will meet at the end of this journey, is Certified Personal Trainer Charles Harris. Charles has been a Personal Trainer for over 15 years. He worked with me years ago to perfect my weight. His special techniques and approach to weight loss have helped women of all ages to accomplish and maintain the bodies they desire. His approach to weight loss is both innovative and pragmatic.

As women, we may get older, but I believe that like a bottle of fine wine, we should just get better with time.

I am so glad that you decided to take this journey with me. Now fasten your seatbelt and enjoy the ride.

## *Fasten Your Seatbelt*

What are your weight loss goals? Write down your weight loss goals for the next 30-60-90 days. If you are like me and try to stay away from the scale, write down your size goal. If you are a size 16, then your goal may be to fit into a size 14 in 60 days. If you prefer to track your success by inches, take your hip and waist measurements. The important thing is to write down your goals. Please make sure that your goals are realistic. Write down your goals; and let's work on making them a reality.

_____

_____

_____

_____

_____

_____

_____

_____

_____

_____

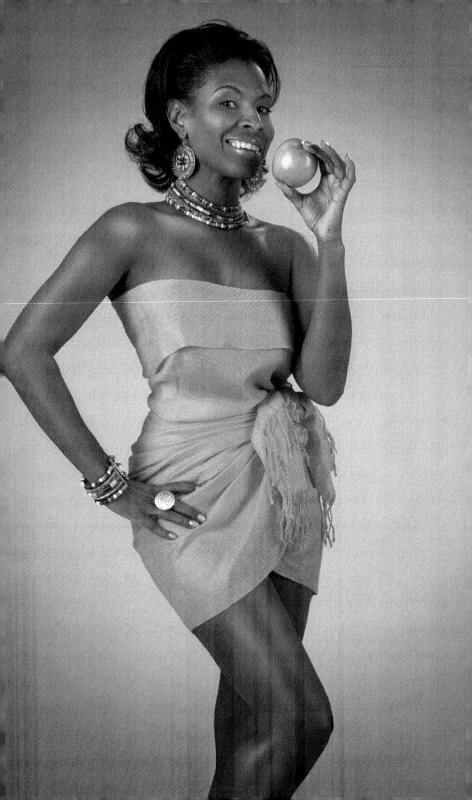

## *Forbidden Fruit*

It's amazing to me that most of the problems that we as women have in our lives—are a result of one woman—the original woman—Eve. Women have not changed much since the creation of the original woman. Eve was a snooper, and women today are still snooping. Okay, you may not snoop in The Garden, but let your man put his phone down for one minute. Let the snooping begin. Eve was snooping in The Garden. She ate the forbidden fruit, and that started our tribulation with food.

So, ladies, don't feel guilty. You are not responsible for your predicament with food. Maybe it's a woman's nature to be curious. But this one is not your fault. It all started with Eve in The Garden. Eve has cursed us again!

When Eve was in The Garden, she was there with Adam, the original man, and the Serpent.

> It all started with Eve in The Garden. Eve has cursed us again!

God told Adam and Eve that they could eat from any tree in The Garden except the tree in the middle. The tree in the middle was a fruit tree (not an apple tree), The Tree of Knowledge. They were warned that if they ate from that tree, there would be a price to pay. Adam, being the obedient one, did not desire to eat from The Tree. But Eve, with her woman's intuition, went against God's word—sound familiar?

Then, Eve did what women do today. She fed the unhealthy, off-limits food to her husband. You do it all the time. You know the food is no good for you, but not only do you eat it, you feed it to your husband and your children as well. Yes, I am pointing the finger at you. I am not guilty of this one. I don't have anything in my house you have to feed or take care of—a man, a pet, a child, or a plant (smile).

I guess misery loves company, and since you know you're going to end up with some health issues, you've decided to take your family along for the ride. You know, you should really be locked up for manslaughter—just kidding!

When God found out that Adam and Eve had eaten from the forbidden tree, he was livid and cursed them. He told the Serpent, "You will wallow on your belly all the days of your life." To Adam he said, "You will toil from sunup to sundown. You will work for the rest of your life." To Eve God said, "You will desire your husband, and he will be master over you. You will have pain during childbirth." And, last but not least, she was told, "You will be ashamed of your nakedness!"

*How many of us are ashamed of our nakedness because of something we ate that was forbidden?*

Wow! That is so profound! I actually came across this passage one year after I started writing this book. It is right there in the Bible. How many of us are ashamed of our nakedness because of something we ate that was forbidden? We ate something that we had no business eating. We read the warning label but decided to partake anyway.

Like Eve in The Garden, we eat things every day that we know will do us harm. And, like Eve, we are paying the price. Eve paid the price back then, and we pay an even higher price today. The price we pay now is high blood pressure, high cholesterol, obesity, and loneliness. I know that many overweight women may get upset by me saying this, but I believe that many women become obese because of loneliness, and many women become lonely because of obesity. We will discuss this in a later chapter.

As soon as Eve ate The Forbidden Fruit, the next thing she did was grab a fig leaf. The Bible says she grabbed the leaf because she realized she was naked. I want to believe that she grabbed the fig leaf not because she realized she was naked, but because she was "ASHAMED" of her nakedness.

How many of us are ashamed of our nakedness because of something we ate that was forbidden? We ate something that we had no business eating. We ate something with a warning label. We, like Eve in The Garden, eat things every day that we know will do us harm. And, like Eve, we cover up with a fig leaf so no one will see our Nakedness. We wear baggy clothes, and when we go to the beach, we make sure we have a cover-up. We hide our bodies because we are ashamed.

When we have sex with our husband, we hide under the covers, all because we did not heed the warning.

I believe that we should start to once again embrace our Nakedness. Naked is the original form in which God presented Man and Woman. The Bible does not say that Adam and Eve were in The Garden in turtlenecks and True Religion Jeans. The Bible says that they were in The Garden Naked. Naked is the original form in which God created all of us.

My wish is that by the time you finish this book, you will no longer desire the forbidden fruit. You will only desire to eat from The Tree of Knowledge. I want you to be able to embrace your body no matter what your size or shape is. But, last but not least, I hope to break the curse left by our sister, Eve, so you will be Naked—and Not Ashamed.

## *Forbidden Fruit*

We all eat something on a daily basis that we know will do us harm. Like Eve in The Garden, we are deceived by the look and packaging of many of the foods we eat. They look good to us, but they are not for us. What are you eating on a regular basis that is deceiving you? You have read the warning label but you still partake. What is your forbidden fruit? Write down your forbidden fruit and what you will do to eliminate it.

_____

_____

_____

_____

_____

_____

_____

_____

_____

_____

_____

_____

## Real Estate

In my 30s, I was a Real Estate Agent. When it comes to a woman's body, I look at it as a piece of Real Estate. Real estate is a valuable asset. It is personal property. Do you believe that your body is a valuable asset? It's God's temple, right? As a piece of real estate, your ultimate goal is to come off of the market, correct? Come on, ladies; you know that your ultimate desire is to use your sex appeal to attract Mr. Right to at least do a walk-through of the property (dating), that leads to a contract (engagement), and then go to settlement (marriage), and live happily ever after!

Notice that I said we use our physical attraction to "attract" Mr. Right. I did not say we use our physical attraction to go out and find Mr. Right. I said we use our physical attraction to "attract" Mr. Right. That's right, ladies, you should not be out looking for a man. The Bible says, "Ye that finds a wife finds a good thing." Not, "Ye that finds a husband . . ." That tells me that the husband is supposed to find his wife, not vice versa. But that's a subject for another book. Let me get back to my point. Okay, as I was saying, your body is a piece of real estate. Let me walk you through the process.

If your body is a piece of real estate, then that means it's a valuable asset. A buyer comes along (Mr. Right) and likes what he sees. The next thing he does is put a contract on the property (he asks you to be his girl.) Afterward, he starts securing the financing, and, in the midst, he's observing his investment. He's checking out how much you eat, how much you make, if you work out, etc. You see, he's evaluating his ROI (Return On Investment). I don't know any investor who's going to invest in anything that will not appreciate in value—do you?

The next thing that happens is the "home inspection." This is the point where the buyer checks out the roof, the electrical system, and last but not least, he checks out the pipes and the plumbing. It's up to you to decide if you'll have your plumbing inspected before closing. I would "highly" advise against it! (smile)

Then, there is the appraisal. This is when the bank confirms that the property is worth the asking price. If the property does not appraise, the bank will not fund the transaction and the property cannot go to settlement.

There are reasons other than the appraisal that some pieces of real estate never make it to closing. One of the main reasons is, like many of us, many properties cannot pass the "home inspection." We don't take care of ourselves, or our bodies, so we have become that undervalued, dilapidated piece of property.

> If you were a piece of Real Estate, would you make it to settlement?

Take the test. If you were a piece of Real Estate—would you make it to settlement? Or would you be put back on the market because your roof is leaking (your weave is bad); you have electrical problems (you have no energy), or your plumbing is stopped up (you have not been to the bathroom in a week because of your poor diet and nutrition.)

Do you know anybody who really wants to invest in a piece of dilapidated real estate?

Start today to increase your own property value. Take pride in yourself. Make yourself a piece of Prime Real Estate. Go through your own home inspection. What's your appraised value? Are you worth your asking price?

It's time for you to make a decision to increase your property value so that you can go to closing and not end up like millions of undervalued real estate today—in foreclosure. I know you can do it......... I'll see you at settlement!

## *Real Estate*

Can you pass a home inspection? Is your roof leaking? Is your electrical system in proper working order? How is your plumbing? Pretend that you are a home inspector. Perform your own home inspection. What do you need to fix to achieve your appraised value? Write down the problems with your systems (include your digestive, circulatory systems, etc.) What will you do to get them in proper working order to be approved for settlement?

_____

_____

_____

_____

_____

_____

_____

_____

_____

_____

_____

## You Must Break Up With Ben and Jerry

Ladies, the first thing you're going to have to do to start living a healthy life is break up with your boyfriends. Don't tell me you don't know who I'm talking about. You know exactly who I'm talking about. I'm talking about the two bad boys you crawl into bed with every night—Ben and Jerry.

When my girlfriend first told me that she was going to bed with three men every night, I thought she was a little kinky, and then she explained to me that the three men she sleeps with are her husband and Ben and Jerry. That darn Ben and Jerry. These guys are wreaking havoc on relationships all over the world. If you are on the road to weight loss freedom, you must break up with Ben and Jerry.

If you are dating these two dudes, you must dump them immediately. I'm warning you; you're in a very abusive relationship, and these guys are no good for you!

I know it's going to be hard to initiate this breakup. You've probably been in this relationship for a very long time. But you must end it right now. They are possibly in your home as we speak. If they are, don't procrastinate. Put the book down, and put them out immediately and promise to never let them back in again. Please make that promise to yourself, because these guys are armed and extremely dangerous!

Oh, and let me warn you; Ben and Jerry have many accomplices! They go by their street names for "credibility." You know them as New York Super Fudge, Rocky Road, and Chunky Monkey. Ben and Jerry hang out with some other Fugitives as well. Have you met Baskin-Robbins? And then there's their cousin Breyers, and who can forget that foreign dude, Häagen-Dazs. These guys prey on beautiful women. They have many pseudonyms, but no matter what they call themselves, they are still accomplices to the two playboys—Ben and Jerry.

If you feel that it's going to be too hard to call this relationship off, then try breaking it off slowly. Instead of dating them in the late hours of the night, start entertaining them only during the day, maybe at lunch. Their damage will still be bad, but not as bad as when you indulge them at nine, ten, or eleven o'clock at night.

> Being with Ben and Jerry is like having a one-night stand.

I have a very close friend named Jan. She is a beautiful woman, very successful, and much sought after in her field. She is in her mid-40s and is a perfect size 8. I keep telling her that if she'd break up with Ben and Jerry that she would be a perfect size 6. She agrees with me and told me that she has tried to end the relationship because she hates herself after each encounter. "Being with Ben and Jerry is like having a one-night stand," she said. "I feel great while we're in the act, but I hate myself the morning after."

If you're in a relationship with any of these guys, then you must do it—you must break it off immediately. Put them out and make sure you put their clothes out with them. You know what I'm talking about. I'm talking about the fudge, the strawberries, the cherries, the wet walnuts, and the things they brought with them to keep them warm and covered at night. Throw it all out with them—now!

The next time you are lonely for Ben and Jerry, try their arch rivals instead, Dannon or Yoplait. If you want an exotic date, take a banana, some strawberries, light yogurt, some ice, and put it all in a blender. Blend it until it reaches your desired consistency and drink it with a straw. It tastes great and is good for you. These guys are much better lovers than Ben and Jerry. They will comfort you and help you forget about the two bums you just broke up with.

I know you're probably asking yourself how I know so much about these guys. Well, I guess I must tell you the truth. You see, I was a victim just like you. I like Hispanic guys, so I had a relationship with none other than Cherry Garcia!

Let me tell you how it started. I was home alone one night and feeling a little lonely, and I remembered my girlfriend, Joan, telling me how great Cherry Garcia made her feel. I also remembered her telling me that I could find him at the corner store. Now, girlfriends don't usually share boyfriends, but Cherry Garcia was an exception, and I was lonely.

As I said I was lonely, so I put on my clothes and got in my car. It was 10:00 P.M.; I drove to the corner store to see if I could find Cherry Garcia. To my misfortune, he was there. I felt bad. I knew I was betraying my girlfriend, but I had to experience Cherry Garcia for myself.

He didn't drive (like most no-good men). So he jumped in the car with me, and we drove straight to my house. Now don't judge me. I usually don't bring strange men home with me. But, like I told you earlier, this was an exception.

When we arrived at my home, I took a shower, changed into something comfortable, turned on the television, lit the fireplace, and slipped into bed with Cherry Garcia.

Ladies, I couldn't believe it. The encounter was unbelievable. He was all over me—my lips—my hips—my tongue—my mouth. I was in heaven. He was the best lover I had ever had. We made insatiable love the entire night. It was one of the best experiences of my life. That's the good news.

The bad news is that it became an addictive

relationship. I knew I was addicted because I had to have him every night. Not only that, but I found myself leaving my home at all times of the night to go get my lover—Cherry Garcia.

One night, I was so desperate that I went to pick him up in my night clothes. That's when I knew I was addicted. Look, don't judge me. I know you have been there before. It's late at night; you're in bed, and you get that strong craving, and usually it's for something that's not good for you. You're too tired to put on your clothes. You put on your coat over your pajamas, put on your slippers, put a scarf on your head, rush out the door, and hope you don't run into anybody you know. That's when you know you're addicted.

The relationship became so unhealthy that I knew I had to end it. I first knew I was in trouble when I started gaining weight like crazy. You know how you get when you're in love. I gained 10 pounds during the first two weeks of the relationship. That was not a good sign. I knew I was in an unhealthy relationship.

One night, I decided not to go pick up Cherry Garcia from the corner store. I was trying to get him out of my system. It was driving me crazy. I was trying to do anything to keep from jumping in the car and picking up my Lover.

Have you ever been there? You're trying to end a relationship but you can't get him off your mind. You have to stay busy. I was doing everything to keep my mind off of him. I cleaned; I cooked; I read anything to clear my head. It worked until I got into bed. I laid there but couldn't go to sleep. My mind went right to Cherry Garcia.

I missed him so much. This was where we shared our intimate moments. And the truth was, I was rarely used to sleeping alone. I was used to having him beside me. I became restless, so I got up and called  my best friend, Karen.

I called Karen and we began to chat. We always talked late at night, and she always made me laugh. We were very close, and she was always very supportive. We all have a girlfriend like Karen; the one that you tell all of your business to. I call them "Flat tire friends." The one you can call at 3 o'clock in the morning when you have a flat tire and you know she'll be there. If you don't have one, you better get one. Flat tire friends are the best.

I had told Karen all about Cherry Garcia,

but for some reason, she never approved of the relationship. She was happy when I told her that we were through, and I was calling her to take my mind off of him.

We were having a great conversation until I heard her laughing and cackling to herself—or so I thought. When I asked her what was wrong, she abruptly told me that she was tired and had to go! I then asked her, "Are you home alone?" She was silent. She then admitted that she had something to tell me—and she hoped I wouldn't get upset. She said she was not home alone. What she said next was like a knife going through my back. She then told me (her best friend) that she was not home alone but that she was there—in bed—with *my* Lover—*Cherry Garcia!*

What? How could this be? How could they do this to me? I was devastated. He had made me feel like I was the only one. And she was my best friend. I should have known better though, because you know what they say: "If they cheat with you, they will cheat on you." And never tell your girlfriends how your man makes you feel. I was devastated! I had been betrayed! I was a victim!

To make a long story short, the bottom line

is, I was in a relationship with Cherry Garcia; I turned into a Chunky Monkey, and it's been a Rocky Road ever since!

So, ladies, if you're in a relationship with Ben and Jerry, please dump them immediately. Because if you're in a relationship with Ben and Jerry—you're in a ménage à trois...and every woman deserves a monogamous relationship!

## *You Must Break Up With Ben and Jerry*

Okay, be honest. Are you one of the many ladies having an affair with Ben and Jerry? Are you part of the harem? If not Ben and Jerry, then what is your late-night indulgence? What is that comfort food that you grab after 9 at night and make love to, that makes you feel comforted, sexy, and satisfied? You know that late-night treat is no good for you, so get rid of it today. What is your late-night indulgence, and what will you do to eliminate it?

_____

_____

_____

_____

_____

_____

_____

_____

_____

_____

_____

## Body Love

Why is it that, as women, we don't take care of ourselves? Women, we are nurturers by nature. Because this is our nature, we spend all of our time loving and nurturing others, but we don't allot the time needed to take care of ourselves. We nurture our parents; we love our boyfriends and husbands; we love our children; we even take care of the dog and the cat. We take care of everyone but ourselves.

Some of you are saying that raising kids and taking care of your family does not give you enough time to exercise and live a healthy lifestyle. But if you want to be around for the kids and other loved ones, you have to find a way to get in shape and practice a healthy lifestyle. In the words of

Oprah, "You must live your best life now!"

When you love something, you take care of it. Don't you love You? So why don't you take better care of yourself? Why are you overweight? Why is your cholesterol high? Why are you a borderline diabetic? You must ask yourself these questions and start taking care of the temple that God has given you. Please remember that obesity has a lot to do with health disparities. You must get in shape now.

> Your body is not a car; you cannot trade it in for a newer model.

Think about it. The body you are in is the only one you will ever have. You will never have another one. Your body is not a car; you cannot trade it in for a newer model. But you can put it in the repair shop (the gym) to get the dings (the fat) out. The mere fact that you are reading this book may be proof that you are not truly happy with your body's composition.

Let me ask you a question. What part of your body are you most in love with? Can you even answer this question? Probably not, because you have not set your eyes on these body parts in a long time. If you only mention your facial features, that is a problem. You should love the muscles in your legs, the firmness of your thighs, the cleavage in your breasts, the bone in the spine of your back, the muscles in your stomach, and the curves of your hips.

I realize that the average woman only spends a limited amount of time in the nude each day. If you are like me, then you're really only nude twice a day—when you shower in the morning and when you shower at night. For those of you who only shower once a day, your nude time is even more limited and your body might be a little tart as well! (smile)

Let me ask you another question. When was the last time you admired yourself in the nude? Yes, that's what I asked you. When was the last time you stood in front of the mirror Naked and embraced You? It's been awhile, so why not do it now. I need you to do it now. Take your clothes off, then stand in front of the mirror and look at yourself. I don't mean just stand in front of the mirror and look. I want you to embrace yourself. I want you to fully embrace You!

Are you happy with the vision? Is it hard

to really look at yourself in the nude? Are you enjoying the experience, or are you embarrassed and unhappy with what you see? Wouldn't it be great if you were in love with your body?

Now that you have embraced yourself, let's identify the areas that you are not satisfied with. Is your midsection a little large? Are your thighs larger than you like? Would you like to lift your breasts? The first step in body rehab is to identify the problem. In the words of Suze Orman, "We can't erase it if we can't face it." Your body is your Picasso! I believe that you are the Architect of your body. Even though Eve started our battle with food, you still have the final word on your Picasso.

Research has shown that your perception of your body can affect your self-esteem. Some women have low self-esteem because they are overweight. On the other hand, some women are overweight because they have low self-esteem. You see, the two go hand in hand.

If you are single, it is even more important for you to be in shape. In his book, *Act Like a Lady, Think Like a Man*, my friend, Steve Harvey, says, "Men are attracted first to what they see." They don't care anything about your dreams, your goals, or your admirations. You will attract men because of your physical appearance—period! You may retain them with your Ph.D., but you will attract them with that nice and firm—well, you know what I'm saying.

Oh, don't get me wrong. I am in no way saying that you have to be skinny to be sexy and attractive. Beauty comes in all sizes, but Healthiness does not. Even if you are a pleasingly plump woman, you can still get in shape, love your body, and tighten it up! As my pleasingly plump sister, Mya, says, "I can't stand a big, fat, sloppy girl, because she makes me look bad."

Something else that you may compromise when you don't love and take care of your body are your intimate relationships. I don't know about you, but I think intimacy is very important in a relationship. I did not say "sex." I said "intimacy." There is a difference. Most people think that sex is more important but intimacy may be just as important, because if you don't have intimacy, you'll never have sex! That's why it amazes me when I hear women say that they are no longer intimate with their significant other because of their insecurity with their bodies. Some of them say that they don't want to be touched by their partners. Women have told me they make love to their husbands in the dark because they do not want their partners to see their bodies. They stay under the covers so that they are not seen in the nude.

That is insane! Ladies, this goes against everything we know about men. Didn't Steve Harvey tell you that men are visual? They want to see you! Imagine how uninhibited you would be if you were not ashamed of your God-given beauty and your God-given body. Imagine if you embraced every God-given curve. You would look at yourself a lot differently.

One area of your body that you must pay extra attention to is your midsection. A U.S. study has shown that women with larger bellies have a shorter life expectancy than women with smaller midsections. The study showed that even though being fat was a problem, more important than that was where the fat was distributed. Too much fat in the abdominal area spells double trouble. Did you know that there is something called "Abdominal Obesity"? You are abdominally obese if your waistline is over 35 inches! Get your tape measure and measure your waistline—

NOW! Don't be afraid! Or just look down at your stomach. Does it look too big to you? If it looks too big—then it probably is. If that measurement is over 35 inches, then you have taken significant years off of your life.

Okay, ladies, if you don't have a tape measure, I will give you another test. If you look down and cannot see the fur on your Cat Box—(you know what I am talking about)—then you have a problem. Your stomach is too big and you are too fat. "Fat" is a word.

> If you can't bend over and see your Va-J-J, that's a problem.

It's in the dictionary. Stop being defensive! Please don't have a Dr. Phil moment on me. I'm going to give you tough love so that you can start living a healthy, productive life and be around to buy my second book (smile).

As I was saying, if you can't bend over and see your Va-J-J, that's a problem. Ladies, your Va-J-J gets lonely, too. Don't you think she would be happy if you would bend down, look her in the eye, and say hello every now and then? You need love, and Va-J-J needs love, too!

Let's get into more details about the abdominal area. Abdominal health is very important for optimum body health. There are two types of fat in your abdominal area: subcutaneous fat (this is the fat that covers your abs) and visceral fat (this fat is within your body and around your organs.) Too much visceral fat is very dangerous because it lies deep in the abdomen; it surrounds your organs and restricts blood flow.

Research has shown that too much fat in the abdominal area is said to be a precursor to Type 2 diabetes. It raises cholesterol levels and promotes insulin resistance. If you have a large midsection, then you are more prone to heart disease, stroke, and breast cancer. Did you know that sleep apnea and migraines have been linked to abdominal obesity?

To live a longer and more productive life, try to keep your midsection as healthy as possible. Pay extra attention to your abdominal area, because excessive abdominal fat is very dangerous. Keep track of your abdominal measurement. And if your midsection is unusually large (over 35 inches), as I told you earlier, you're in big trouble. So let's work on reducing it today.

Although it's great to be in shape and to be appealing to the eye, please know that it's also great to be in shape so that you can live a full, productive life! Undoubtedly, the greatest benefits to being in shape are the health benefits.

Today is the first day of the rest of your life. Remember, it's hard to find someone to love you if you don't love yourself. Love yourself and your body enough to get in shape, because obesity can kill your self-esteem and confidence—and it may one day kill *you*! Commit to start practicing Body Love Today!

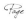

## *Body Love*

We should all love our bodies. Take your clothes off, stand in front of a mirror and write down three parts of your body that you are most in love with. Now, write down the parts of your body that you are least in love with. What are you willing to do to improve the areas that you are least happy with so you can fall in love with your body again? Remember, it's important to love the skin that you're in, so write a love letter to yourself and discover everything you love—about You!

_____

_____

_____

_____

_____

_____

_____

_____

_____

_____

_____

_____

## What's Eating You?

Studies have shown that many times people are not obese because of what they are eating; most people are obese because of "what's eating them." There are many reasons why people eat emotionally. Some people eat because they are bored. Some people eat because they are lonely. And there are some people who just like to eat! We all know and accept drug addiction and drug abuse as problems in our society. But few know that there is another type of addiction that goes unnoticed. That addiction is called "Food Addiction."

> I define food addiction as the "continuous abuse of food."

I define food addiction as the "continuous abuse of food." This abuse is real and goes undetected on many occasions. Just like with any other form of addiction, the first step in any treatment program is first admitting that you have a problem. You must diagnose yourself and be self-aware.

If you find yourself eating all day long for no reason at all, and it sounds like I'm talking to you—I need you to repeat after me: *Hello, my name is _____, and I am a food addict.* Okay, now that you have confessed your addiction, let the recovery begin.

My girlfriend, Kym, is a real food addict. Her full name is Kymberli Pinkard and she lives in Austin, Texas. That's right, I put her entire name out there, because we must do an intervention. If you see Kym, please don't give her any food; instead, give her a hug and let her know you read about her in my book (smile). Kym describes food the way a woman describes a man she just met. My girlfriend pines for food the way a woman pines for love. She says that she feels aroused by the anticipation of food. Kym says she salivates; her heart palpitates when she has a delicious meal. She intakes food with all her senses. Kym is in a "bona fide" love relationship with food that surpasses any logical reasoning or understanding. Plain and simple—Kym is a Food Addict!

Kym eats because she's a food addict. Why do you eat? Do you eat because you are hungry, or do you eat because something is eating you?

I have another girlfriend who eats ice cream and cake like nobody's business. She's celibate. I believe that eating sweets is orgasmic for her. I promise you that every time she eats sweets, she experiences a climax of some sort. You cannot tell me any different! You should see the look on her face when she indulges in sweets. It's X-rated! I told her that she has made eating sweets her personal sexual experience. What's eating her is her inability to express herself sexually. So she eats to replace her sexual void, and even though she's not horribly obese, I told her if she keeps eating aggressively, she soon will be.

I have another girlfriend who has never dealt with the death of her father. So she eats when she starts thinking about and missing her dad. She eats to fill a void of abandonment.

There are many reasons why people eat that

have nothing to do with hunger. Some women eat when they end a relationship. They eat to fill a void of loneliness. I've never understood that philosophy; when I end a relationship, the last thing I want to do is eat. More than food, I'm concentrating on being my best so I can look good for the next Romeo who might come my way.

Another reason you don't want to eat after a breakup is because when your "ex" sees you again, you want him to say, "Wow!"—not "Dang, she looks a hot mess!" After a breakup, overeating is the worst thing you can do, Every diva knows that looking good is always the best revenge!

We fill many voids in our life with food. We sometimes try to control stress and anxiety with food. So the next time you start to binge eat, ask yourself: "Am I really hungry, or am I trying to fill a void?" Is something eating you?

If you're overweight or morbidly obese, it's very important that you ask yourself "Why?" It's important that you get to the root of the problem. And let me tell you now, you may not be able to solve your problems alone. You may have to confide in your spouse, a friend, your pastor, or someone else that you trust because this may prove to be a hard journey to take alone.

You may even have to seek some professional help (psychologist) for healing. Don't be afraid of the couch, ladies. You have been on the couch before, for less appropriate reasons (smile). Now, it's time to lie on the couch to heal the pain. Who knows, the psychologist may be a stud. Use whatever means necessary to get to the root of the problem. You must figure out what's eating you so that you can live a healthier, happier, more productive life.

So the lesson here is—to remember: Your weight gain may not be a result of what you're eating; it may be a result of what's eating you!

## *What's Eating You?*

Have you ever stopped to really think about the reason for your weight challenges? Is it the boyfriend you lost? Is it the stress from your job? Are your children stressing you out? Is your marriage going through challenges? It may not be what you're eating; it may be what's eating you. What's eating you? Take a moment and write down the top reasons for your challenges with your weight. If there are health issues, then please let's pray for healing. If there are other reasons, then please take a moment and write down those reasons so that we can let the healing begin.

_____

_____

_____

_____

_____

_____

_____

_____

_____

_____

## You Are What You Eat

How many times have you heard the phrase "You are what you eat"? If this is true, then we are in some major trouble. If that is true, then I'm in trouble because I'm a slice of pizza with green peppers and jalapenos or a piece of birthday cake.

What does it really mean? What does your diet say about you? Let's think about this. It means that if you eat beef, then that would make you a cow. What woman wants to be a cow? If you eat pork, then that would make you a pig. That's not sexy at all. And if you eat chicken, that would make you one of the ugliest creatures on the face of this Earth. Who wants to look like a chicken?

A friend of mine and I have a game that we

love to play. We look at people and name them after the food that they reminded us of. For instance, my chubby sister, Mya, reminds me of a delicious cheesesteak submarine with everything. My girlfriend Dina is caramel-colored and really sweet, and she reminds me of a stack of pancakes with pecan syrup. I have another friend who looks so unhealthy that she looks like a hot dog with chili—and that's not cute at all! I have another friend who is always swollen because of an unhealthy diet and all of the Martinis she drinks. I promise you—she looks like a pork chop smothered with gravy! I have another friend who is so unhealthy that she reminds me of a sausage.

> You can look at someone and can tell that they have an unhealthy diet.

Now, I will never reveal their names, but my point is, I believe that hardly anyone looks like anything healthy!

Have you ever noticed that you can look at some people and can tell that they smoke or drink? I don't know what it is, but they have that unhealthy look. I believe the same is true about food. You can look at someone and tell that they have an unhealthy diet. It especially shows in their skin. What about those coffee drinkers? Why is it that most coffee drinkers do not have white teeth? Could it be that coffee stains them?

"WHAT DO PEOPLE SEE WHEN THEY SEE ME?" What would you like for them to see? I know for me, instead of looking like a piece of pizza or a piece of birthday cake, I would prefer to look like strawberries or blueberries; something sexy, colorful, healthy, and sweet.

Start making smarter food choices today. I guarantee your appearance will represent a healthier lifestyle. So, next time you decide to indulge in something unhealthy, please remember—You are what you eat!

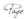

## *You Are What You Eat*

We all agree that we have heard the saying, "You are what you eat!" If this is true, then what are you? What do people see when they see you? Do people see something good, or do they see bad food choices? Are you a cow, a banana, a hamburger, a bagel, or ice cream, etc.? Write down your results, and if it's not a healthy representation of you, then let's make more nutritional food choices. Write down what people see when they see you and then write down what you would like for them to see.

_____

_____

_____

_____

_____

_____

_____

_____

_____

_____

_____

# Eat Your Food Naked

This is the chapter you've been waiting for: Eat Your Food Naked. Like I said before, I don't want you to just take your clothes off, get a plate, put it in the microwave, and have a meal. There is more to the title than that.

When I first told my girlfriend about the title of my book, she called me the next morning and said, "Girl, I ate my food naked last night, but when I sat down at the table and saw my stomach sitting on my lap, I didn't eat as much." All I could say was—"MISSION ACCOMPLISHED!"

My girlfriend, Cheryl Jackson, said that if she ate her food naked, by the time she looked at all of her fat rolls, she would probably never eat again. My girlfriends have taken the test; now it's your turn. I want you to take the test—see how you feel about your body when you eat your food while naked. Yes, now it's your turn. I'm asking you to "Eat your food naked!" I want you to take all of your clothes off, go fix yourself a plate—and Eat Your Food Naked.

How did you feel when you were eating your food Naked? Did you feel uncomfortable? Could you see your Va-J-J? Was your stomach in your lap? Did you eat as much? Were the rolls on your sides larger than the rolls on your dinner plate? If they were, then you're in big trouble!

Like I mentioned before, when I came up with the premise for this book, I was not only talking about you getting naked, but I was also talking about the actual food that you eat—eating that naked as well.

I know what you are thinking: *How do you eat food naked?* When I say, "Eat Your Food Naked," that means I want you to eat your food in its rarest form. Let me help you understand. Some foods are born naked, and they are great. Carrots, pickles, nuts, cucumbers, celery, tomatoes, apples, oranges (fruits), and broccoli—these foods should make up the majority of your diet.

There are some foods that are not naked that

you can make naked. Let me give you an example. If you're having chicken, take the skin off. Having a salad? Skip the croutons, feta cheese, and cranberries. Salads seem to be a healthy choice but can sometimes be very unhealthy—by the time all of the extras are added: the nuts, the strawberries, bacon, and the salad dressing. You might as well have a submarine sandwich.

Try eating your salad naked—with only vegetables and a small amount of salad dressing. Eat your salad with lettuce, tomato, celery, cucumbers, and a pinch of fat-free dressing. Keep the salad a healthy meal as it was meant to be. Eat your food without all the "dressings" and extras that we pour on that make it an unhealthy choice. These add major calories and no added nutritional value.

So, imagine what would happen if you ate most of your food naked. The cheeseburger without the bun; the French fries without the chili; the hotdog without the works—get the picture?

Okay, I know that for some, maybe most of you, this is a radical change. You may not have the self-control or discipline you need to eat your food completely naked, so let's start by eating your food semi-nude. Start by taking off one slice of bread on your sandwich. Start by eliminating one fattening item from your salad. Start by taking off one item at a time until your food choice is completely nude.

When you order a pizza (if you really need to indulge), how about ordering a thin-crust pizza with one topping instead of a pizza with everything? Eat your pizza "Naked."

Speaking of pizza, I always say that when you order a plain pizza, it still comes with two toppings. They give you one topping for free—the extra grease! With as much grease that drips from the pizza, they really should count that as a topping! A good tip: Always blot your pizza with a paper napkin to remove the excess grease from the cheese. You'll eliminate lots of unwanted calories.

There is a national food chain that sells Naked Tacos—a taco without the shell. By eliminating the shell, the taco is naked—and healthier. You still get the lettuce, tomato, protein—everything that is healthy. But you leave off the fattening taco shell. Oh, and whatever you do, please don't eat the fattening guacamole!

The opposite of eating your food naked is eating your food with everything. And that's the problem—nothing you eat should come with everything. It drives me crazy when people order hotdogs and sandwiches with "everything" or "the works." Half the time, no one knows what "everything" or "the works" even includes. They're just being greedy. If you find yourself ordering your food, with everything or "the works," that's a red flag. You're in big trouble!

Let me help you start eating your food "Naked." Here are a few more examples: Instead of eating a baked potato overloaded with butter, sour cream, chives, and cheese, eat the baked potato naked. It may be too harsh to put nothing on the potato, so try it partially nude, with only a little salt, pepper and some I Can't Believe It's Not Butter! It tastes so good, you'll believe it is.

> I think it's sexy when you "eat your food naked."

If you're one of those people who has to eat a bagel every morning (which is the worst thing you can put in your body), please don't eat the bagel with cream cheese. Eat the bagel plain. Why are you eating bagels anyway? Did you know that one bagel can be the equivalent to 3 to 4 pieces of

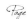

bread? If you must eat a bagel, please eat it naked.

You have to start somewhere! I think it's sexy when you "eat your food naked." You must get rid of the extra toppings. Remember a minute on the lips, forever on your hips! So, start eating your food naked so you'll be happy when you eat your food naked—and be Naked and Not Ashamed.

## *Eat Your Food Naked*

How will you begin to Eat Your Food Naked? What will you take off that pizza? Will you eat your sandwich with one slice of bread, or will you wrap it in lettuce? If you must eat chicken, will you remove the skin? What will you eliminate from your favorite dish to make that dish a healthier choice? Write down five things you will do to begin to eat your food naked or partially nude.

_____

_____

_____

_____

_____

_____

_____

_____

_____

_____

_____

_____

_____

## The "F" Word

The "F" word. I know what you're thinking, but as a virtuous woman, I "try" not to curse. The "F" word is usually a bad word, but in this case, it's not. In this case, when I talk about the "F" word, I am speaking about one of the best things a woman can put into her body, and that is Fruit.

Consuming fruit is essential to any healthy weight loss plan. I love fruit. But what I find is that most people drink their fruit instead of eat it. If you want an orange, then eat an orange instead of drinking orange juice. If you want some grapes, eat some grapes instead of drinking grape juice. If you have a taste for pineapple, eat a pineapple instead of drinking pineapple juice. Get my drift? Most fruit juices are full of sugar and are no good for you. You must eliminate juice from your diet immediately. Juice is just as dangerous as soda. The only time I drink juice is at communion. I love that Welch's grape juice (smile).

I think many of us don't eat fruit because we are bored with it. But why not try eating fruits that are as sexy as you are? I like apples and oranges, but I love more exotic fruit. I eat mangoes, pineapples, apricots, and pomegranates. The next time you go to the grocery store, walk past the boring fruit and try something more exotic. I think you will love your new choices.

Some research suggests that MS, Alzheimer's, and Parkinson's disease can be prevented by adding more fruits and vegetables to your diet. These diseases may be caused by poor dietary choices. What's so interesting is that some researchers believe that not any fruit will do. Some research has shown that purple fruits may have more health benefits because they have properties that may protect the brain cells and they are also full of antioxidants.

You are now asking yourself, *What are antioxidants?* I know you've been hearing that word thrown all around, but nobody has taken the time to explain to you exactly what they are. Antioxidants are nutrients that are found in food that can slow down the oxidative damage to your body by neutralizing free radicals. Antioxidants are also said to slow down the aging process. Sign me up!

Okay, let me break it down. We are exposed to free radicals throughout our lives through sun exposure and environmental pollution, as well as internally through alcohol consumption, smoking, unhealthy diet, etc. When our body's cells use oxygen, they also produce free radicals that can cause cell damage and lead to chronic diseases. Many scientists agree that free radical damage is the major cause of degenerative conditions and aging. Antioxidants repair the damage done by free radicals. Thus, diseases such as cancer and heart disease, to name a few, may be avoided.

> Antioxidants repair the damage done by free radicals.

Since we are exposed to free radicals every day, I believe it's important that we get our proper supply of antioxidants to help us repair the damage done to our bodies.

ᴊome fruits that are high in antioxidants are pomegranates, prunes, strawberries, blueberries, cherries, raspberries, plums, and kiwi. Do your research and you will be amazed by the benefits of antioxidants.

I said earlier to try to stay away from fruit juices laden with sugar, but there are some juices that are healthy for you; I'm talking about juices that are supplements.

I drink a juice every day that is full of antioxidants. The juice that I drink is called Le'Vive. This juice has Noni, Goji, Mangosteen, Pomegranate, and Acai all in one bottle. Before I started drinking this drink, I would be very sluggish, but after drinking the drink for about a week, the results were dramatic. I had so much energy—it was unbelievable. It also curbed my appetite.

The testimonies about this drink are astounding. There are testimonies from lowering high blood pressure to healing of joint and muscle pains. I find Le'Vive to be a great appetite suppressant. I can't live without my Le'Vive or my antioxidants. Please try to include more antioxidants and fruits to your diet. And don't forget melons; they are also great fruit selections.

Oh, and one more thing, please don't be like my sister. I called her one night and asked her what she was doing. She told me she was eating, and I asked her what she was eating at 10 o'clock at night. She told me to calm down; she was eating fruit. Okay—now, I know Mya, and there was no way she was eating fruit at 10:00 p.m. (She had just broken up with her boyfriend, too, so I knew she needed comfort food.) I asked, "Mya, what kind of fruit are you eating?" She started laughing hysterically and finally blurted out, "Apple pie!" Ladies, a slice of apple pie does not count as a fruit serving! So, the next time someone makes you mad and you want to curse them out, instead of using the "F" word—pause and put a piece of fruit in your mouth instead. And please don't forget— no apple pie—because you must "Eat Your Fruit Naked!"

## The "F" Word

Fruit was the first food given to man. However, I believe it's one of the healthier foods that we have abandoned. Most fruits are high in antioxidants and are essential to a healthy diet. We know that berries are high in iron and antioxidants. We should try to consume at least 2 servings of fruit a day. Eating 2 servings a day will really help bowel regularity. Do you consume fruit on a daily basis? If not, what fruit will you include in your diet immediately as part of your lifestyle change? If you already eat fruit, what exotic fruit will you add to your diet? Please record your plan below.

_____

_____

_____

_____

_____

_____

_____

_____

_____

_____

## *Sugar Mama*

If you find yourself in bed with Ben and Jerry, you just might be a Sugar Mama. Many women are Sugar Mamas. That doesn't mean that you take care of a man the way a Sugar Daddy takes care of a woman. In this instance, a Sugar Mama is a woman who is addicted to Sugar. How would I know? I know because I'm a Sugar Mama. I have to have my Sugar. I can't stand those diets that tell you to eliminate all sugar. To me, that's not logical. Why should I deprive myself of life's little pleasures? I believe "There's no bad food—just bad portions."

We all have our sweets of choice—for me it's birthday cake and Baby Ruth candy bars. It may sound real crazy, but I love birthday cake, and, guess what, as I said earlier I don't deprive myself of what I like. I have a fresh piece every week, usually from the local grocery store. (Safeway's is the best!) Notice I said I have a piece a week, not a piece a day.

I used to be so bad that during my stint as a Real Estate Agent, one of my investors, Julius, used to bring me a whole birthday cake to every settlement. I would eat a small piece of cake at the office. But one thing that I would never do is bring that cake home with me. I would always leave that cake right in my office—out of sight, out of mind.

> I believe you should treat your sweets like you treat your men; never bring temptation home with you!

I believe you should treat your sweets like you treat your men. Never bring temptation home with you; never let it cross your doorstep!

It may be hard not to be a Sugar Mama, but I think you will feel better as a Healthy Mama. The first thing you should know about sweets is that if you have to indulge, only have a small portion. When I am eating anything sweet, three is the magic number. I never have more than three bites!

In three bites, I have usually satisfied my craving.

Another thing I do when I am eating something sweet is that I savor every bite. I consume it slowly; I enjoy each and every second and each and every bite. I try to do this with whatever I'm eating. The slower I eat, the less I consume. I also find it healthful to put my fork down periodically when I eat. Have you noticed we never put our forks down between bites anymore? We eat as if we're in some type of race. Your brain needs a minute to get the message that you're full.

Now, while I know that you may not be ready to totally eliminate all sugar from your diet, you can certainly cut back a bit. If you are a cookie monster, buy the mini bite-sized ones instead of the regular cookies. I love the mini Oreo Bites. If I must indulge, I usually eat about three to four little minis in one sitting, and my sweet craving is usually satisfied.

For those of you who feel like being real warriors and want to eliminate sugar from you diets altogether, I suggest purchasing sugar-free items. Walmart has an entire section of sugar-free candies. You can also purchase sugar-free gum, ice cream, and cake. Because we are trying to be a more health-conscious society, food companies are providing just about anything that you can think of as a sugar-free option.

Please remember when reading labels that carbohydrates are sugar!

Some of you may be saying, "I don't eat a lot of sweets; that's not my weakness," yet, you drink two Pepsis a day. By the way, you know you're addicted to sodas when you start hiding them around the house from the rest of your family. You hide them because you have to have that fix there when you are ready for it or you'll go into withdrawals. If you fit into this category, then you're one of the millions of people who drink their calories instead of eating them.

I have a small challenge for you. Eliminate sodas from your diet for one week, and then take note of the change in your body. You should give up sodas altogether and substitute soda for water. If you can't substitute regular soda for water, then substitute it for tea, or diet soda, or anything but regular soda.

If you're walking around looking like you're six months' pregnant, it may be from the three sodas you consume every day. Please get rid of all soda in your diet. It's no good for you; it has no nutritional value, and it's making you fat. I guarantee that you'll see a difference in your midsection in about ten days.

Some of you are probably saying that you don't have a problem with sweets and you don't drink sodas. Well, what about the orange juice you consume daily? Do you realize how much sugar is in orange juice? Have you ever wondered why the orange juice glass is the smallest glass on a hospital tray? I can tell you why—it's because orange juice is full of sugar!

Did you know that sugar stores itself in your midsection? If you want to get rid of that belly fat, start by getting rid of the sugar. My trainer told me that sugar sits in your midsection and your midsection is controlled 70% by diet, 20% by nutrition and 10% by rest.

So, ladies, cut back on the sweets; eat smaller portions; share if you can, and eat your sweets during the day if you must indulge. No matter how many crunches you do, if you don't eliminate most sugar from your diet, it will be hard to get that body you desire. Try to cut back on sweets as much as you can, and the next time you want to overindulge, please remember—Nothing tastes as good as looking good—Nothing!

## Sugar Mama

Are you a Sugar Mama or a Healthy Mama? Are you addicted to sugar? Please write down what sugar you consume on a regular basis. Are you addicted to birthday cake like me? Is it candy? Is it ice cream? Is it soda? Is it bread? Please remember that bread is a carbohydrate that turns to sugar in your body. Write down the sugar that you will attempt to eliminate from your diet. What healthy choice will you substitute it with?

_____

_____

_____

_____

_____

_____

_____

_____

_____

_____

_____

_____

## I Think I'll Have a Happy Meal

Ithink I'll have a Happy Meal. I know you are asking yourself, *What in the world is she talking about?* What I want to talk about in this chapter is portion control. It has been said that portion control may be the single most effective way to promote and maintain lasting weight loss.

I believe that you can get in shape and not deprive yourself of life's natural pleasures. This can all be done by exercising portion control. In my world there is no bad food, just bad portions.

Portion control has been one of the biggest contributors to my weight maintenance. I believe you can have anything you desire—in moderation. We talked earlier, in the chapter with sweets, about smaller portions. When I have a craving for birthday cake, I will never buy the whole cake—just a single slice. And then, I'll take that slice and cut it into two separate slices. You see—it's all about portion control.

When I want a candy bar, instead of buying one large one, I'll buy the bags that are usually sold around Halloween—you know, the bag with the miniature candy bars. I'll eat one (sometimes two) candy bars, and my craving is satisfied. This concept can be used for all meals.

The title for this chapter came about because my sister and I were at McDonald's one day, and, of course, I ordered the salad with light dressing. But my sister, Mya, ordered a Big Mac, a large fries, and a large milkshake.

I said, "Mya, do you know how many carbohydrates you're about to eat? And then, you'll be complaining to me about how fat you feel and how you can't lose any weight." Mya really thinks she's funny. She looked at me and said, "Are you finished scolding? Because, on that note, I think I'll have two Big Macs, two large fries, and a super-sized drink."

So we went back and forth for about five minutes, and, finally, she looked at me and said,

"Okay, you're right. I get what you're saying. I'll get what I want—just a smaller portion." Then she said, "Come to think of it, I'll have a Happy Meal!"

I loved it. That was the beginning of a (small) change for Mya. She was full from the Happy Meal. And what do you know, she never ordered another regular meal in my presence again!

If I ate meat, I would definitely order Happy Meals. I love the toys that come with them (smile). They really come in handy at children's birthday parties. And if you become really bored, they can entertain you.

When I was a Flight Attendant, I would always order off the children's room service menu on my layover. Don't knock it until you try it. Oh, one thing I have to tell you: If you're going to do this, remember that before they bring your food up, you have to run the shower in the bathroom and close the door so they'll think there's a child staying in the room. You have to do this because I got busted once. They brought my food up, didn't see a child in the room, and charged me full price! I found a way around that though; now I stage a child's presence every time. I order off of the children's menu. I bet they'll never get me again!

I was amazed to find that there was a study conducted sometime ago that analyzed the eating habits of French women. What was interesting about the study was that it revealed that the French women ate pasta and bread and consumed alcohol, but never gained weight. The secret to their noticeably small frames was the portions that they consumed. Their portion sizes were considerably smaller than the portions of American women. The French ate pretty much whatever they desired, but only in moderation.

> The only way you can get a small portion nowadays is to order a kid's meal.

There are a couple of ways to ensure portion control. One way that you can ensure proper portion control is by never eating on a full-size plate. In my house, all of my plates are the size of saucers. I can only eat what's on the plate. If it won't fit on the plate, there's a good chance that it will not go into my mouth! Try this in your home. It will make a big difference.

If you constantly eat out, this portion control battle isn't going to be an easy one. Everything today in the U.S. is super-sized. The medium cups are large, and the large cups are extra large. The only way you can get a small portion nowadays— is to order a kid's meal.

Let me ask you this: As parents, why do we not insist that kids order off of the kid's menu? Is there something wrong with a child eating a child's portion? I can never understand why parents won't let children order off the kid's menu. This blows my mind. I have a girlfriend who never orders off of the children's menu for her daughter, because she says her daughter eats more than a child's portion.

That's the problem! Her daughter is eating more than a child's portion, and it shows. She's as big as a house! The crazy part is that my friend should be able to see this for herself. The child is already suffering from low self-esteem. I'm sure that her classmates tease her. Kids aren't kind to other kids who are fat. The child is 15 to 20 pounds overweight and is probably suffering from childhood obesity. And her mother monitors nothing that she eats.

That reminds me, I was out once with a girlfriend and her daughter. We were at a restaurant with an extensive children's menu. But instead of the mother insisting that the child order her breakfast from the children's menu, she let the child order from the regular menu. I couldn't believe it. This 12-year-old child sat in front of me and ordered a Breakfast Sampler and a large orange juice. Do you know what came on that sampler? Let me tell you. I want you to visualize a 12-year-old eating this—two eggs, two pancakes, two pieces of sausage, turkey bacon and two pieces of toast, and that wonderful drink that passes itself off as healthy—orange juice.

I watched this precious child and realized that we are digging our children's graves with a knife and fork. Childhood obesity usually leads to obesity as an adult, and that can be dangerous and lead to an early death. It is very important that we teach our children about nutrition and portion control at an early age. Studies have shown that if you are obese as a child, you will most likely be an obese adult.

More than likely, if your Mama's fat, you'll be fat. But I don't believe that fat is hereditary. Most of the time you become fat from EATING TOO MUCH! As I said before my Mama is a size 20 something. But Mama can eat! She did not inherit a dang thing. She earned every pound.

We must break the generational curse of bad nutrition in our families. I have chosen to start with me.

Remember, there are no bad foods—just bad portions. Practicing portion control will really help you maintain or obtain that hourglass figure. Portions are so large now that one meal can usually feed two to three people so try to share your food whenever you can.

Speaking of large portions. Look at The Cheesecake Factory. I love that place, and I don't deprive myself. When I treat myself to The Cheesecake Factory, I will usually order a salad and have an appetizer as my main course (Firecracker Salmon Rolls). If I want to treat myself to a entrée, I insist on sharing my entrée with whomever I am dining. If I have dessert, I ask that they cut one piece of cheesecake into two slices, before they bring it to the table. It's always more than enough.

When my girlfriend, Dina, and I go out, it's an unspoken word. We order two salads. We share an entrée, and we share dessert. It works every time and it's more economical. You have to admit, when you are out with your girlfriends, it's really

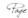

not about the food. The restaurant makes it about the food, but that's really not what's important to us. To us it's about the ambiance and the bonding experience.

While paying attention to your portions, please try to wean yourself off of fast-food. Eating fast-food in your car can be so unsanitary. When you eat fast-food, you're usually eating with your hands. Your hands are usually dirty, because they have been on your steering wheel, on your cell phone, on bathroom doors, in your hair, up your nose, scratching your butt. Do you get my drift? Your hands are filthy! When you eat fast-food, nearly everything that goes into your mouth has been touched by your hands.

Sounds like another reason to stay away from fast-food. But if you can't totally walk away from fast-food completely, the next time you have that craving, walk up to that counter, lift your head, and with confidence, proudly declare to the cashier—"I think I'll have a Happy Meal!"

## *I Think I'll Have a Happy Meal*

You may not want to go through the drive-thru and order a Happy Meal, but what process will you implement to ensure smaller portions? I firmly believe that portion control is essential for weight maintenance. What is your commitment to portion control? Will you commit to eating on smaller plates? Will you commit to eliminating the word "large" from your vocabulary when ordering consumables? Will you commit to sharing your dessert? Write down your commitment to ensuring proper portion control.

_____

_____

_____

_____

_____

_____

_____

_____

_____

_____

_____

Page

## Don't Be a Lemon

Ladies, have you ever had one of those days when you just wake up on the wrong side of the bed and act like a sour lemon all day? Well, the next time this happens, don't be a lemon; try sucking a lemon instead. Did you know that lemons are one of the most important fruits created by nature and should be a very important part of your diet!

Lemons have been used in Chinese medicine for years. Known to be a good source of vitamin C, they have been linked to reducing the risk of cancer and are thought to also prevent heart disease. Lemons contain fiber, potassium, and thiamin. Thiamin is

> Lemons have been used in Chinese medicine for years.

important because it helps the body convert carbohydrates to energy and helps improve brain and muscle function. Niacin helps lower LDL (bad cholesterol) and raises HDL (good cholesterol).

Have you ever seen people who suck on lemons and thought they were doing it because they liked the way the lemons tasted? Well, although there are some who love the taste, lemons have a plethora of healthy benefits.

Here are a few:

*Lemons are used to cleanse the mouth.*
*Lemons can relieve constipation.*
*Lemons help improve digestion.*
*Lemons can be used to eliminate parasites in the body.*
*Lemons can be used to reduce gas.*
*Lemons can prevent urinary tract infections.*
*Lemons are used to relieve rheumatic pain.*
*Lemons are used to combat sore throats and asthma.*
*Lemons have antibacterial properties that are good for healing wounds.*
*Lemons can be used to remove free radicals from the body.*
*Lemons can be used to help lose weight.*

Lemon water also has many health benefits. If you are a coffee drinker, put the coffee down and try some lemon water in the morning instead. After dinner, skip the coffee; order lukewarm lemon water. It's a known fact that coffee will dehydrate your body, but lemon water will hydrate your body.

It is great to start your day with lemon H20 since lemons are a natural diuretic. Here are some of the benefits of drinking lemon water:

*Lemon H20 is a blood purifier.*
*Lemon H20 is great for digestive support.*
*Lemon H20 helps fight fatigue.*
*Lemon H20 boosts your metabolism.*
*Lemon H20 strengthens the liver functions.*
*Lemon H20 may help dissolve gallstones.*
*Lemon H20 is great for your hair and your skin.*
*Lemon H20 cleanses and detoxifies the body.*

Lemon water is great, but I never drink lemon water away from home unless I have my own lemons. The reason for this is quite simple. The 2007 *Journal of Environmental Health Study* showed that when seventy slices of lemons were collected from over twenty different restaurants, contamination was found on most of the lemons.

This is not hard to believe. The contamination could have come from unclean work stations or from the hands of the employees. I don't know,

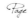

I can only imagine. It kills me when I'm with someone and they order a drink and ask the bartender or waiter for a lemon. That is the most unsanitary thing in the restaurant.

You know they cut the lemon, and squeeze it into your drink with their dirty hands—Yuk! That is nasty! Where have their hands been? Studies show most people don't wash their hands after they use the bathroom, and ladies, we all know that many men have a bad habit of scratching their testicles. I don't think I want those unclean hands to squeeze my lemon!

One of my girlfriends told me that there were actual feces found on lemons from one study—that is disgusting. We don't need to go into much detail about that. But please, try not to eat any lemons in restaurants; only use lemons that you have brought with you. It may not be classy to pull a lemon from out of your purse, but it will definitely be more sanitary! No, just kidding. Don't put a lemon in your purse, but you can carry that little lemon-shaped container of lemon juice in your purse to spruce up your drink.

I believe that lemons should be a major part of your diet. Truly, lemons are a necessity. One precaution before I end this chapter: If you choose to suck lemons, don't suck too many, because they have lots of acid and that can ruin your tooth enamel.

So try adding lemons to your diet. I think you will love the results. Sugary lemonade does not count! So the next time you want to be a lemon, eat a lemon instead—you will be a lot healthier, and your friends will be a lot happier—I guarantee it!

## Don't Be a Lemon

As we discussed earlier, lemons are a very important fruit for a healthy body. Lemons have many medicinal effects and are a great source of vitamin C. Lemon water aids the digestive system, can act as a blood purifier and helps promote weight loss. Are lemons a part of your diet? What will you do to make lemons a part of a healthier lifestyle? Will you substitute the coffee that you drink in the morning that dehydrates you—with warm lemon water to hydrate and cleanse you? Please write your plan below.

_____

_____

_____

_____

_____

_____

_____

_____

_____

_____

_____

## *Animal Racism*

If we don't eat dogs, then why do we eat chickens? This has always intrigued me. I, myself, am not a meat eater (it's a personal choice) but I do indulge in chicken maybe once a week. I am trying to eliminate chicken from my diet completely, and, thank God, I'm almost there. I am not trying to be Vegan, but I am trying to be Veganish.

Now, I'm not trying to get into trouble like Oprah did with cattle ranchers, but I challenge you to do your own research on chicken, beef, and pork, and ask yourself if meat is something you really want in your body? Better yet, since I know you are busy, go to YouTube and watch one of the vid-

> If we don't eat dogs and cats, why do we eat chickens?

eos of cows being slaughtered, or watch a video of a chicken farm. I think that may help you decide how much meat and poultry you want to consume.

Did you know there was something called mechanically separated poultry (MSP) and mechanically separated meat (MSM)? This is when a machine cleans the meat off of the animal's bones. You see, the animal owners want to make sure they get every scrap off the animal's bones, so they put it in a machine. In the case of poultry, when it comes out of the machine, it comes out looking like pink paste, so it has to be dyed. Maybe that's the blood from the animal; I don't know. Oh, and it has lots of bacteria, so it has to be soaked in ammonia to remove the bacteria. Oh, and one more thing; it tastes really bad, so it has to be reflavored to have the taste of chicken that you're used to. All of this so it can make it to the food supply and be delivered to your dinner table as a healthy meal—Yummy!

Did you know that many store-bought brands of Chicken McNuggets are made of mechanically separated poultry? Some sausage, bologna, and hotdogs are also produced using this process. Start reading the labels. It has become recent law that mechanically separated meat and poultry must be labeled as such.

Okay, back to my point. It's hard trying to write a book with ADHD (You know the HD stands for high-definition—smile!) If we don't eat dogs and cats, why do we eat chickens? And after what I just told you, why do we eat any of it? Why is one species of animals treated more sacred than others?

Let's start by looking at the way we treat dogs in America: We buy them clothes, give them their own homes (a dog house), have their nails polished, take them to the doctor (the veterinarian), take them with us on vacation, take them to have their hair done (grooming), and allow them to sleep with us (not me—the only dog I want sleeping with me is a man— oops!) They now even have their own hotels and playgrounds. We treat dogs and cats sometimes like royalty. We sometimes actually treat some of them better than we treat our own children. Why is it that we are so in love with dogs and cats? You can even go to jail and serve time for abusing them.

But then, on the other hand, you can actually murder some animals and there are no consequences to pay! Wow—that is pretty profound. You can kill a cow, kill a chicken, kill a turkey, and a Presidential candidate can make a sport out of shooting geese, and there are no consequences! But if you abuse a dog, you have hell to pay! You don't even have to kill a dog; just give someone the idea that you are abusing them, and you may have to answer to charges of animal cruelty. Just ask Michael Vick.

There was a newscaster who said that Michael Vick should be executed for taking part in a dogfighting scandal. Give me a break! Now don't get me wrong, I believe that what Michael Vick did was wrong, but you can commit mass murder and not be executed.

People love dogs and cats but continue to abuse other species of animals. What is that all about? What does this say about us? Could this be a sign of Animal Racism?

I BELIEVE THAT ANIMALS ARE ANIMALS—LIKE HUMANS ARE HUMANS. Cows and chickens have breath and breathe life just like dogs and cats. They breathe and bleed the same, but why do we favor one species over the other?

If you look at a cow, the cow usually is brown or black. Could it be that the cow is the Negro of the animal race? The cow is usually hung by its neck and tortured before death. Does that sound familiar? This sounds a little like the abuse of a race of people that I am quite familiar with. The cow is to the animal race what the African-American was to the human race. They are hung, abused, and tortured the same way!

I have an idea: Let's try to end Animal Racism. Let's commit to treating all animals the same. Let's stop eating animals. Who said we need to eat animals to live? I don't think so! Let's make a commitment today to not eat anything that bleeds or breathes. Come on, you can do it—Try not to eat meat every day. Wean yourself off slowly. Cut your meat intake down to 3-4 times a week until you completely eliminate it. Try it—not only will you be saving animals' lives, you will also feel much better.

> Could it be that the cow is the Negro of the animal race?

I'm committed to ending Animal Racism—What about you? I hope you stand by me with my commitment! We must stop eating animals. I'm committed—but I tell you—I'm sure gonna miss that fried chicken—Cluck, Cluck! (smile)

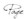

## *Animal Racism*

Do you believe there is something called Animal Racism? What four-legged animals do you consume on a daily basis? Are you a racist? Do you love dogs and cats but continue to consume cows, pigs, and chickens? What is your commitment to eliminate or cut back on eating anything that breathes or bleeds? How do you intend to end Animal Racism?

_____

_____

_____

_____

_____

_____

_____

_____

_____

_____

_____

_____

_____

_____

## Fake It 'Til You Make It

D id you know that you can reshape your body with reshaping garments? Did you know that there is something called the Science of Reshaping? Do you believe that you can drop 2 to 3 dress sizes in 10 minutes without diet, pills or exercise? I did not believe it either until somebody introduced me to this garment called the Body Magic.

The Body Magic is one of over twenty reshaping garments designed by Orthopedist Leonel Kelly Mexia through a company called Ardyss International. Ardyss International is a Health and Wellness company out of Mexico that specializes in reshaping garments for men and women. The garments deliver orthopedic benefits but are comfortable to wear. Reshaping garments take inches off of your body instantly and give you a smooth foundation in your clothes. I have been wearing the garments for over two years now, and I love them.

Some of the garments that the company manufactures include the corsets, corselettes, reshapers (short, lightweight body suits), high-waisted girdles, and T-shirts for women that remove those rolls on the side when you wear tight shirts. They also manufacture postpartum and maternity girdles. Oh, one other thing before I move on: This company does not discriminate. Ladies, we all know that there are many men walking around looking like they are about three to four months' pregnant. My girlfriend and I have a joke that when men constantly wear big shirts on the outside of their pants, they are probably suffering from "Dunlap Disease." His stomach dun lapped over his belt (smile). Does your man suffer from Dunlap Disease? If he does, you may want to purchase two garments: one for you, and one for him. I don't know about you, but I am an equal opportunity employer, so I want my man's body to look just as good as mine. I don't think we should give them a pass. I believe it's time to start holding men responsible for their bodies as well.

The garment that Ardyss International is most popular for is called the Body Magic. Many celebrities wear this garment to achieve an hourglass figure and to help with weight loss. The garment is like a one-piece full girdle, but it is not a girdle. It reminds me of half of a body suit. It is like a modern-age corset that covers the hips and the midsection. The Body Magic is an innovative creation that will transform your body, and give you an immediate hourglass figure.

The Body Magic lifts, shifts, and gifts. It lifts the breasts, giving the appearance of an instant breast lift. It flattens and controls the abdomen muscles, giving the appearance of liposuction without surgery, and it gifts the buttocks by lifting and rounding the buttocks area while thinning the thigh and hip area. The garment redistributes the fat from where it is (where it should not be) to where it is supposed to be. Fat should only be in two places—the buttocks and the breasts—and the Body Magic helps you accomplish that goal.

The first time I saw the garment, I was at a Showcase. They asked for a volunteer, and a woman came to the front of the room. They took a measuring

5

tape and measured her waist and thighs. Her waist was 41 inches and her hips were 50 inches. They took her to a dressing room and put her in a Body Magic. When she returned to the front of the room, the transformation was unbelievable! She looked amazing. Her measurements were taken again. Her waist was reduced to 38 inches and her hips were reduced to 46 inches. The biggest change, however, was in her self-esteem. Her self-esteem went through the roof—and her smile was priceless!

**The panty reshaper locks the gluteus maximus into its proper position!**

What I like about the garment is that once a woman puts the garment on, she can see how she will look once she reaches her desired weight goal. I believe that many women may need this experience. We are a microwave society, and we like immediate results. The Body Magic delivers on this request.

There are many reshaping garments, but another one that really intrigued me was the garment that gives you the appearance of a larger derriere. This garment is also manufactured by Ardyss International and is called the panty reshaper. This garment is unbelievable. The first time you see the garment it will blow your mind. It is the craziest-looking garment that I have ever seen. It is like a pair of underwear with a hole cut out in the buttocks area. Did you know that without the assistance of reshaping garments, the buttocks begin to shift downward? The panty reshaper locks the gluteus maximus into its proper position! By using the reshaping garments, you maintain the original shape of the buttocks. This garment helps to give you instant buttocks and helps eliminate irregularities in your hips and thighs by taking the extra tissue from the hips and thighs and redistributing it to the buttocks. With the panty reshaper garment, every woman can be "Bootylicious"!

I love my reshaping garments. They have actually aided in reshaping my body. They have become like The American Express Card. I can't leave home without them.

As I said earlier, you do not want to wear the Body Magic forever. I believe that you get into that garment to get out of it. Once you reach your desired weight, there is no need for the Body Magic again. There may not be a reason for a Body

Magic; however, I strongly believe that reshaping garment should always be a part of every woman's arsenal.

The minimal use of a reshaping garments is one of the reasons why so many of us are walking around obese and out of shape. Women have abandoned undergarments. I know we wear brassieres and underwear (some of us anyway), but that's it.

What happened to those girdles our mothers used to wear? I remember my mother struggling every morning to get in her girdle. How can I forget that? I helped her on many occasions. When did we get away from this? It's funny; in those days it was a girdle and a wig! They went together like peanut butter and jelly. I am glad we got rid of the wigs, but, ladies, we must bring the undergarments back!

I often wondered how the ladies of the early years on television maintained their hourglass figures. Now I know their secret. It was with reshaping or foundation garments. These ladies wore corselettes, girdles, or something to maintain their sexy, girly figures.

So much has changed. Today, women walk around with fat all over the place, and they don't even care. I hate to say it, but it disgusts me. Women today no longer walk around with hourglass figures; they walk around nowadays looking like—football practice dummies. It's ridiculous!

There is no reason to walk around with your stomach hanging over your belt, when we now have garments that can take care of that appearance. Ladies, if you see rolls on your side in your clothing, that's a problem. Rolls should only be served at the dinner table with butter. Get rid of those rolls with a nice corselette or corset. What do you think those celebrities you see on television are wearing? The secret's out! If you took some of those celebrities out of their reshaping garments, I promise you, it would be a hot mess!

Reshaping garments are great, not only because many of them actually reshape your body, but because they also give you a smooth foundation in your clothing. So, ladies, until you totally create the body that you desire, order a few reshaping garments—and fake it 'til you make it!

## *Fake It 'Til You Make It*

We all have areas of our body that we are unhappy with. If you are like me, I am impatient and need immediate results. What reshaping garment will you commit to wearing to give you those immediate results while you work toward making them permanent with proper nutrition and exercise? Will it be a girdle, corset, or corselette? Remember the correct combination of garments can give you an immediate hourglass figure. Write down two reshaping garments that you will commit to wearing as you work toward creating that beautiful body!

_____

_____

_____

_____

_____

_____

_____

_____

_____

_____

Eat Your Food NAKED

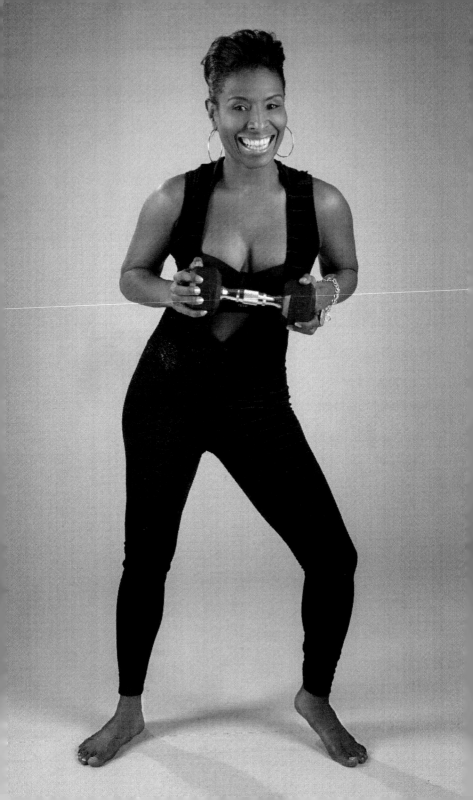

## *The O Workout*

We can wear all of the reshaping garments we want, but we will not achieve our ultimate goal without a good diet and exercise. As we get older, it sometimes becomes harder to work out. We have children and husbands (sometimes these are one and the same), aging parents, demanding jobs, etc. With all of these obligations, it sometimes becomes impossible to find the time to pack a bag and make it to the gym to have an effective workout. We use our busy schedule as a reason not to get the daily exercise that a healthy lifestyle requires.

The media has fooled us into believing that we must go to the gym to get an effective workout. I don't believe this is true. Although, if you have the time, going to the gym and working out with a trainer is a great way to ensure that you get the proper workout your body requires. But many people don't have the time to fit this into their daily routines.

I have found that there are many exercises you can perform right in the comfort of your own home, or if you travel as much as I do, they can be performed in your hotel room. When I became very busy and was unable to make it to the gym to work out because of travel, or to be honest, a lack of motivation, I had to find a way to incorporate a workout into my daily routine without leaving home.

I started doing what I now call the "Oprah Workout." This is a workout that I now do as I watch Oprah. Yours may not be called the "Oprah Workout," but name it after the favorite show that you rush home to see almost every day. I don't care if it's a sitcom, a soap opera, or the news. Name your workout after the one television show that you never want to miss.

The first thing you must do is get all of the equipment that's in your exercise room or in your basement and move it to your bedroom. I started by moving my stationary bike, dumbbells, stability ball, and bands to my bedroom, in front of my television. You may not have that much equipment, but whatever you have, get the dust off of it and move it into your bedroom.

Now let me tell you how the Oprah Workout goes. Okay, you are sitting there watching Oprah, but as soon as there is a commercial, you must get on (or pick up) a piece of workout equipment; or if you have no equipment, you must do some type of exercise during the entire commercial. It can be jumping rope, jumping jacks, running in place, push-ups, or anything that exerts energy. This is great for people who are a little rusty. You will only be doing 3-4 minutes of exercise with this process per commercial. This will equal about 15 minutes of cardio for the hour. This can be a lot for someone who has not exercised in a while. This will help you begin to increase your stamina, which is a very important step toward increasing your heart rate and getting ready for a regular workout regimen. It's hard to believe but many people who have never exercised will feel a change in their energy level just from exercising during the commercials of their favorite television show.

But it doesn't stop there. That is the first baby step. After you become comfortable with this format, and you have an increase in energy, then you must change the game a bit. What I want you to do now is the opposite of what you did in the beginning. I now want you to exercise during your favorite show and take a break during the commercials. That should allow you about 45 minutes of cardio a day. That's a major switch, don't you think? This process will allow you to commit to almost an hour of cardio a day—without leaving home.

If you can't follow this plan, at least try to do 20 minutes of cardio every day. We all know how important cardio is. Cardio helps to increase your heart rate for a period of time, which helps you burn fat. Cardio also helps you increase the rate in which you burn calories. When your heart is pumping faster, you increase the number of calories that you burn.

> The goal is to get at least 20 minutes of cardio every day.

It's great if you can do your cardio in the morning so that you can get your heart pumping early. Running is a great cardiovascular exercise. You don't have to be on a treadmill or at an outdoor track to run. When you're on a treadmill, you're going nowhere and that drives me crazy. You can run in place in front of the TV if you like, run up and down your steps; get that heart pumping any way you can.

If you travel a lot, as I do, you don't need to find a gym. Many exercises can be performed in your hotel room with no equipment. You can do push-ups, sit-ups, jumping jacks, lunges etc. So, see you don't need any fancy equipment to start an effective workout regimen. As a matter of fact, you don't need any equipment at all. The only thing you need is your body and the desire to make a change.

Please don't think that you have to invest in a bunch of expensive workout equipment to be in shape. I would advise you to invest in three pieces of equipment for your home workout, if you like. A stability ball, a jump rope, some dumbbells and a hula hoop. I guess that's four pieces of equipment. That's right, a hula hoop. Exercise should be fun. Remember when you used to hula hoop how much fun you used to have. Go and get your hula hoop from the toy store today. It's great for the waistline. You'll love it.

If you want to invest in something that's a little more expensive that the entire family can use, the Wii Fit is a great investment. You can bowl, play tennis, run, hula hoop, etc. The sky's the limit with the Wii Fit.

Let's talk about the pieces of equipment that I mentioned. I love the jump rope because this is a small piece of equipment that you can take with you anywhere you go. With the jump rope, you can start off very slowly and increase your reps. I am not asking you to do the Double Dutch. I am asking you to start by maybe doing 50-100 reps and then increasing that to 2-3 sets of 100 reps, working yourself up to 500 jumps 3-5 days per week. The results will be amazing. Jumping rope gives you a total body workout. If you commit to jumping rope every day, then you will feel great and see immediate results.

Dumbbells are great for women who don't have the time to go to the gym to work out and want to build muscle. I love them because you don't have to exert any energy to use them. If you don't feel like doing cardio, you can sit on the side of the bed and do your tricep and bicep curls while you're watching your favorite show. I will sit on the side of the bed sometimes and continuously do my tricep and bicep curls. I started by doing three reps of 15. That is about 45 reps on each arm. I now try to incorporate 10 reps of 10 as part of my regimen.

What I love about working the arms is that, I believe you can see your results quicker there than any other part of your body. When your arms are sleek, I think it enhances a woman's sex appeal. The results of the bicep and tricep curls are amazing. You will not believe how this exercise can slenderize and give muscle mass to your arms. There is nothing worse than seeing a woman's arms still waving long after she's said goodbye.

While we are speaking about arms, another great exercise is what I call the "kitchen sink push-up." Whenever I'm in the kitchen—and that's not often because I can't cook—when I think about it, I stand in front of the kitchen sink with my body slanted and use the sink to push my body up. Start by doing maybe 10-20 push-ups and work your way up to 50. The results you will see with your upper body will be incredible.

Ladies, if you are walking around with flabby arms, it does not have to be that way. Run out and purchase some dumbbells, or stop by your nearest kitchen sink today!

The stability ball is another piece of equipment that every woman needs in her arsenal. I love the stability ball, because everything you do on this piece of equipment works your core. You can pick up a stability ball up at your nearest sporting goods store, Target, or Walmart. The stability ball comes with an air pump. Blowing up the ball is another form of exercise in itself.

Anything you do on the stability ball will work your core. The core is important; it's where you get your inner strength. It is the inner, most essential part of your body. A strong core helps with injury prevention, posture, and balance. If your core is strong, then your body is probably strong as well.

Charles will give you some exercises for the stability ball later in the book. But let me share with you some of the things that I love about the ball.

What I love about the ball is that even if you just sit on it, you're working your core! You can actually feel your stomach muscles compress by simply trying to balance yourself on the ball.

You can sit on the ball for an hour while watching TV, do leg raises and crunches across the ball, bicep curls, or be creative and invent something yourself! It's that easy. If you're sitting on the ball doing bicep curls, you're still working your core.

You can take the ball, put it over your head, and bend from side to side. You are now working your waistline. If you take the ball over your head and bring it down to your knees and then bring it over your head again while you continuously do these reps, you're also working your core. You should be able to feel the pull in your midsection. It feels amazing.

I don't know why, but exercise gives you an astounding energy boost. Many women have found that when they exercise, they have more energy during the day. It's funny; when I neglect my home exercise routine, I feel very lethargic during the day. But when I exercise, my energy level is greatly increased.

Ladies, before we end this chapter, I would be remissed if I didn't discuss one of the most popular home activities known to man. This activity is, of course—sexual activity. Most of my married girlfriends complain about the sexual relationships between themselves and their spouses. They look at sex as a chore. I am not married, so I don't have to perform that chore. Sex is for married people—right (Biblical)?

Wives, instead of looking at sex as a chore, how about looking at it as recreation? I am sure your husband likes for you to be creative, so what better game to play in the bedroom than to pretend that your mate is an inanimate object? You can pretend that he is a mat. Lay him on the floor and work it out! You can do sit-ups on him, push-ups, or lunges. If you want to be really sexy, you can sit on the mat and do some bicep and tricep curls. If you really want to use the bedroom as your personal gym, grab that kitchen chair and do some leg lifts and push-ups. Of course, all of this is done in the nude with your mate as a spectator!

So, the next time you have relations, don't look at it as a chore, ladies; don't think about your husband and the wrong that he may have done. Remember, "It's all about you" and that gorgeous

> Wives, instead of looking at sex as a chore, how about looking at it as recreation?

body you want to achieve to deny him the next time he's a "bad boy."

Ladies, you know deep down inside we all LOVE a bad boy, so, just because he's bad—doesn't mean "It's" not good. Don't deny yourself. Just because he's naughty—doesn't mean you can't have a smile on your face!

## *The O Workout*

Now that you know that exercise is an essential part of a healthy lifestyle and you don't have to go to the gym to be "Firm and Fabulous," what exercise routines will you commit to, from the comfort of your home? What will become your O Workout? Please write down 3 exercises that you will begin at home and record what time you will perform these exercises on a daily basis or a minimum of 3 times a week. You can keep the bedroom exercises to yourself. That's house business! (smile)

_____

_____

_____

_____

_____

_____

_____

_____

_____

_____

As I was doing research and reading many periodicals for my book, some things blew my mind. As I conversed with many of my friends and family members, they were astounded by some of the information I shared with them. As I said earlier, I am not a workout guru or fitness expert, but like you, I am a woman who wants to look good when she eats her food naked. And since you and I are now friends, there are some things I think you should know.

Did you know that 1 bagel can be the equivalent of 3-5 pieces of bread?

Did you know that some cows are dismembered while alive to be prepared for human consumption?

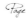

Did you know that an egg is a chicken's fetus?

Did you know that chickens eat stink bugs, worms, etc., and we eat chickens?

Did you know that ham is a pig's BUTT?

Did you know that some studies have shown that eating red meat increases your risk of colon cancer?

Did you know that a study conducted showed that 83% of chickens purchased in stores had some type of bacteria?

Did you know that catfish are bottom feeders and eat any kind of dead fish, rats, etc.?

Did you know that Russian catfish were found with human remains inside them? They do not kill people, but they eat them once they are dead, and we eat catfish.

Did you know that some people eat the viscera intestines of a pig (chitterlings)?

Did you know that Coke and Pepsi can be used to clean car batteries?

Did you know that the healthiest food is usually on the perimeter of the supermarket?

Did you know that some vegetables may protect against colon cancer?

Did you know that adding whipped cream can add 50-100 calories to a beverage?

Did you know that one hush puppy can equal 50-60 calories?

Did you know that usually the more color in a food, the healthier it is for you?

Did you know that pig's hair is sometimes used for brushes?

Did you know that a Caesar salad is usually not a healthy choice, because it comes with croutons and the dressing is made of raw eggs?

Did you know that fruit juice is sometimes added as a sugar to granola?

Did you know that most chicken farms are not inspected?

Did you know that when you eat meat or poultry, you are eating hormones, drugs, and chemicals that were fed to the animals before they were slaughtered?

Did you know that coffee may have a diuretic effect?

Did you know that wine contains some iron?

Did you know that some pigs like to scavenge and that some pigs suffer from influenza?

Did you know that muffins are closer to cake than they are to any healthy choice?

Did you know that icing is made of shortening and sugar?

Did you know that there are very few minerals in some mineral water?

Did you know that some meats are cloned?

Did you know that some tomatoes are ripened by gas?

Did you know that a salad taco shell can equal 300-400 calories?

Did you know that carbohydrates are sugar?

Did you know that breakfast bars are usually very high in carbohydrates?

Did you know that some chickens are given antibiotics to accelerate their growth?

Did you know that pigs have no sweat glands and lie in mud to cool off?

Did you know that many processed foods are derived from corn?

Did you know that many cows are fed corn and not grass to accelerate their growth?

Did you know that counting carbohydrates is as important as counting calories and fat?

Did you know that milk may contribute to mucous?

Did you know that 60-90% of diseases can be prevented by diet?

Did you know that live rodents, mice, and maggots have been found on some chicken farms?

Did you know that salmonella outbreaks sometimes stem from feces?

Did you know that recently, 5-foot-high piles of manure were found on a chicken farm?

Did you know that donuts are fried?

Did you know that meat can give you smelly poop and gas?

Did you know that a pig's bones are sometimes used for glue?

Did you know that drinking 8 glasses of water a day may prevent constipation?

Did you know that sausage may contain some part of a pig's lung?

Did you know that the average American eats around 38 pounds of high fructose corn syrup per year?

Did you know that the average American will eat 36 pigs and over 700 chickens and turkeys during their lifetime?

Did you know that fat-free foods are not always fat-free?

Did you know that some juices have as much sugar as sodas?

Did you know that some batches of high fructose corn syrup, when sampled, were contaminated with mercury?

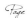

Did you know that I knew you did not know these things—and that's why I am writing this book! (smile)

## The Royal Throne

You may think this chapter is full of crap, and you're right, but we must talk about your bowels and the Royal Throne (toilet). It's a known fact that women don't go to the Royal Throne as much as they should. There was a time when I would only have a movement twice a week. Ladies, if this is you, then this is a very serious problem. It is vital that your food passes through your bowels. People who suffer colon cancer usually have a history of constipation.

Some experts say that you should go to the throne after every meal. Some people say that the definition of a normal bowel movement is having one movement a day. Some experts say that you should go 2-3 times a day, while others say that it is not about the frequency, but that it is about the color and the consistency. There is said to be no rule for frequency, but the general rule is from 3 times a day to 3 times a week. There is so much conflicting information on bowel movements that when I did my research, I did not know which way to go. So, I will discuss the theory that makes sense to me.

I believe, like many experts, that it's not really about the frequency as much as the consistency. Let's talk about the color of your stool. The bile is secreted from the liver, meets the food just past the stomach, and it stains the stool a greenish brown.

That is why your poop is brown. The stool should not be the color of the Cleveland Browns uniform; it should be that magnetic Gucci brown—you know, the color of your favorite Gucci bag, that medium brown, the color of cardboard. If your stool is dark in color, like black, it may be a result of those iron pills that you are taking. But if you're not taking iron pills, it may signify a bleeding stomach ulcer.

Your stool can also be dark because it has been sitting in the intestines for a prolonged period of time. This is a problem. This could signify constipation. You may need to add more fiber to your diet.

Have you noticed that there are sometimes other fluids in the throne with your stool? Have you ever seen the white mucous around your poop and wondered, *What is that?* Well, that mucous may indicate inflammation in the intestines. You also have a higher chance of having mucous in your stool if you're constipated or if you have diarrhea. However, if your stool is all white, there could be a serious problem, and you should see your physician immediately. White stool can signify gallstones, hepatitis, cirrhosis, or maybe even tumors.

Have you ever seen lumps in your stool? Chances are you may have eaten some corn earlier that day. Did you know that your body cannot digest corn? That's a whole 'nother story.

Okay, now let's talk about the time you went to the throne and saw blood with your stool. If you have blood in your stool, there may not be any reason to be alarmed. This may be a result of constipation or inflammation in the intestines. But there may be other reasons for blood in the stool such as ulcers, polyps of the colon, hemorrhoids, cracks in the lining of the anal opening, and maybe even Crohn's disease. If blood in the stool continues for a prolonged period of time, please consult your physician. Dr Oz, my favorite doctor, said that your poop is like a mood ring. And different colors are indications of things going on in the body.

Another thing that's important when we talk about stool is the scent. Notice that I did not say odor (that has such a negative connotation.) Now, I'm not saying your stool should smell like Prada perfume, but it shouldn't smell like rotten eggs or your man's underarms after a workout at the gym either. If you keep air freshener in your bathroom for the aftermath—that's a sign that something's out of order. Poop that leaves a stench is a sign of undigested food and increased fat in your stool and may be an indication of a bad diet!

> Remember, ladies, there should be no straining or discomfort when visiting the throne.

Remember, ladies, there should be no straining or discomfort when visiting the throne. It should be a very uneventful process. Your stool should have the consistency of a gel and should leave your body easily. Your stool should not hit the water like an atomic bomb. It should enter the water smoothly and float to the top gracefully like the Queen that you are.

We cannot conclude this chapter without talking about one of the greatest problems with women—constipation. Constipation is the difficult or incomplete passage of stool. Constipation is usually a result of the lack of fiber. It has been said that you are constipated if you do not go to the throne at least 3 times a day. If you're going to the bathroom less than 3 times a week, if you're straining to go, or if your stool looks like little pellets—you're probably constipated.

Constipation is usually a sign of not enough roughage in the diet. There are many treatments for constipation, many over-the-counter remedies. But since I am against medication, let's talk about some natural ways to solve that problem.

The first thing you can do to combat constipation is to incorporate more fruits, vegetables, and whole grains into your diet. Prunes will also get you moving. There is no better way to start your morning than with a bowl of whole grain cereal or oatmeal with a minimum of 4-5 grams of fiber per serving. Consuming more roughage is also a great way to combat constipation. Please, ladies, eat as many green, leafy vegetables as possible. Remember, the more color in your food, the healthier your diet.

We all know that vegetables are part of a healthy diet, but one of the best ways to combat constipation is by drinking water. Females do not drink enough water. Water should be an essential part of a woman's diet. Water combats constipation, but it's also great for your skin and aids in hair growth. If you are not drinking enough water, you should increase your daily H20 intake immediately. Start your day with a nice, tall glass of water or a small glass of warm water. You will be surprised at the difference this will make in your bathroom consistency and your skin. I try to drink at least 5-6 glasses of water per day.

Ladies, it may not be the sexiest thing to do, but please start to observe your poop and remember; You're a Queen—and every Queen should visit her throne on a consistent basis! (smile)

## *The Royal Throne*

Ladies, I know you don't want to do this, but you have to start taking a look at your stool and taking note of your consistency. Please record how often you go to the Royal Throne on a weekly basis. What color is your stool? Does it have an odor? What shape is your stool? Are you constipated? If you are constipated, then what will you do to repair this problem? Will you add more water to your diet? Will you cleanse your system more? Will you add more roughage to your diet? Please write down your plan.

_____

_____

_____

_____

_____

_____

_____

_____

_____

_____

_____

## Tricks of the Trade

Ladies, thank you for taking the ride with me. I hope you enjoyed the journey. I know I made you laugh but I may have even made you cry. The journey that we took was to get you to this final destination, which is a serious conversation about weight loss. Obesity is killing millions of Americans each year. It has become a national epidemic.

Please remember diets are temporary fixes. What you may need is a lifestyle change. A journey begins with the first step. And you've taken it. You have to have a plan to stay in shape. So please write your plan down today. The Bible says, "Write the vision on the wall."

Being over 40 and still a size 4 is a true blessing. There are some things that I will never do, and there are other things that I will always do. My girlfriend always laughs and calls them "tricks of the trade." I don't know if they are tricks. But here are some practical principles that I have incorporated in my life for years to help me stay in shape.

We covered a lot of information in this book. I would like to do a quick recap with you and maybe share some new tricks with you as well.

As women it's important that we remain Fine, Fit and Fabulous, so please take heed of the Tricks of the Trade.

*-If you must eat a sandwich, always take off the top piece of bread.*
*-If you can eliminate bread altogether, use lettuce as a wrap instead*
*-Always share dessert*
*-Never order a large quantity of anything*
*-Decrease your meat intake to a maximum of once or twice a week*
*-Always blot your pizza to remove the grease*
*-When at dinner never have bread, wine, appetizer and dessert; pick one or two of the four*
*-If you must eat candy, try to substitute it with sugar-free types*
*-Always have the waiter pack one-half of your meal to go*
*-Eat white foods in moderation*
*-Never eat out of containers (you will eat more)*

-Never eat a bagel

-If you may be tempted to eat more than a proper portion of a meal or dessert, pour water in it...it will no longer be desirable

-Remove all unhealthy snacks or sweets from your home

-Try not to eat anything 4 hours before bedtime

-Try to eliminate all soda from your diet

-Try to consume 6-8 glasses of water per day

-Stay away from fried foods

-If you must eat bread, please substitute white bread for wheat bread

-Always eat off of a small plate or saucer

-When you're going to a dinner party, eat before you leave home; that way you are not tempted to overeat

-Please remember that a buffet is different from "all you can eat"

-Give up Martinis (full of sugar)

-Substitute ice cream for sorbet

- Make lettuce the wrapping for your sandwich

-If possible make dinner your last meal of the day

-Always practice portion control

-Eat your food slowly and lay your fork down between each bite

-Instead of eating a baked potato with butter and sour cream, try eating a sweet potato with butter substitute

-Never eat in dim light (you will eat more)

-Remember if it comes in a box, it is probably not good for you

-Never wait until you are hungry to eat

-Remember lunch should be your largest meal (you will have more time to burn off the calories during the day)

-Eliminate fast-food from your diet

-Replace 3 large meals with 4-6 small ones

-Replace drinks high in sugar with water or drinks low in carbohydrates

-Try to make dinner your last meal of the day

-Substitute Stevia and raw honey for sugar

-Incorporate more fruits and vegetables in your diet

-Remember your hunger signs may be signs of thirst— not hunger

-Remember chewing gum (sugarless) can relieve hunger cravings

-Eat vegetables and fruits 2-3 times per day

-Substitute beans for protein instead of meat

-Substitute sandwiches with soups, beans, legumes and salads

-Drink 2 glasses of water in the morning before you eat anything to hydrate your body

-If you don't like the taste of vegetables, add them to a smoothie in the morning; you will get the nutritional value without the taste

-Stay away from coffee; it dehydrates your body, and browns your teeth; substitute it with green tea or lemon water

-If you must eat cereal, make sure that the first ingredient is a whole grain

-Drink lemon water; it's great in the morning as a natural diuretic

-Remember to always eat fruit by itself

-Don't forget to cleanse your body, including your colon

-Substitute regular milk with almond milk

-Always drink water before every meal; you will partake in less calories

-If you have the will power, restrain from eating anything but fruit until noon every day

-Start wearing reshaping garments so that you can see how you will look once you reach your desired results

-Commit to home workouts a minimum of 3 times a week if you cannot make it to the gym

-Stay off the scale and use a tape measure to measure inches lost

-Add antioxidants to your diet

-Eliminate pork from your diet

-Never eat in your car

-Try to make half of every meal vegetables

-Try not to eat on the run

-Don't deprive yourself; take 3 bites of that forbidden food and be done

-Eat your fruits instead of drinking them

-Limit or ELIMINATE your orange juice from your diet (it's full of sugar)

-Always carry healthy snacks with you: nuts, carrots, etc.

*-Always check the serving size on everything you eat and drink. You will be surprised that you are sometimes eating or drinking 2 servings in one sitting. If a container says 2.5 servings per container, 200 calories per serving, and if you drink the entire beverage, you have consumed 500 calories in one sitting.*

Remember…..."Nothing tastes as good as looking good" and don't be afraid to Eat Your Food Naked!

Arrival

Ding…Ding

On behalf of your entire flight crew, we would like to welcome you to the Land of Healthy Living. Please remain firm with your abs tight until the aircraft has come to a complete stop at the gate—and the captain has given you a two-bell signal indicating you are fit enough to stand and move about the cabin. At that time please check underneath your breasts for firmness and in the seatback pocket in front of you for any flab you may have brought onboard.

Use caution when removing sweets from the overhead compartment because cellulite may have shifted during the flight.

Please check the television monitors inside the terminal building for updated exercise classes and nutritional information.

On behalf of your "Alter Ego," we would like to thank you for flying Naked Air.

We appreciate your business and look forward to serving you on a future flight.

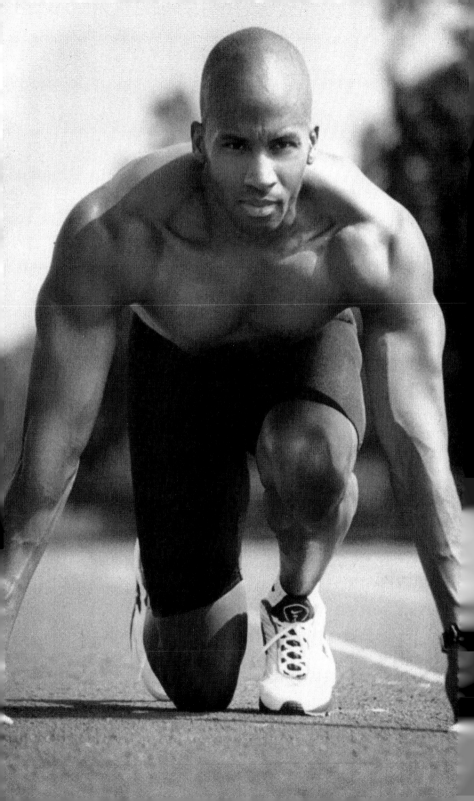

## Charles Harris

Charles Harris is a highly effective fitness and lifestyle coach with a passion for the health and wellness of all humanity. His personal, lifelong battle with high blood pressure became his source of motivation to help others confront and conquer their health issues. In business for over a decade, Charles has been certified through the Aerobic and Fitness Association of America (AFAA), featured on NBC Morning Weekend Fitness, and, most recently, he completed the Iron Man 70.3 Competition. His signature fitness routine, coined "Chizel-It," is a 45-minute workout that combines cardiovascular activity, kickboxing, and strength training. His signature workout caters to all fitness levels and is sweeping the nation.

Through various principles, Charles "Chizel-It" Harris teaches his clients how to live a balanced life of physical, emotional, and spiritual health. Because he believes that nutrition is an integral part of a healthy way of life, Charles focuses his efforts on nutritional training and education that leads to an improved diet, better fitness, and a healthier lifestyle, which leads to a total transformation of the Mind, Spirit, and Body.

## *Affirm Yourself*

Before I start any workout plan with a new client, the first thing that I have them do is Affirm Themselves. We all have a little voice in our heads that says something like, "I can't lose this weight," or "I don't have time to exercise. The minute we start verbalizing our negative thoughts, we automatically set ourselves up for failure. One way to overcome negative speaking is to learn the power of positive affirmation. We need to pay more attention to our thought process in life and this holds true in exercise.

Each time our inner voice starts saying words such as "can't," "try" or "but," we need to verbally overcome those thoughts with a positive affirmation. Positive affirmations are the foundation to achieving our physical, spiritual, and mental goals. For example: if you want to lose 10 pounds in 30 days, don't say, "I want to lose 10 pounds in 30 days." Just say, "I am losing 10 pounds in 30 days!"

Every word we speak, whether positive or negative, has a major impact on our lives. Even when we feel bad physically, we should be saying things like: "I feel young, healthy and strong"; "I have never felt better than I do right now," or "by His stripes I am healed!" You are who you say you are; you can do what you say you can do! Life and death is in the power of the tongue!

> Every word we speak, whether positive or negative, has a major impact on our lives.

## *Let's Get Started*

Now, that you've made the mental commitment to get in shape... let's get started! You can't let the media control your senses or appetite. You should use your eyes to read food labels and see what foods contain high fructose corn syrup and MSG. These ingredients are in 95% of all the processed foods we consume on a daily basis. In some cases these ingredients are impossible to avoid. You must become more knowledgeable of the food that you eat. Make a conscious decision. God's people are destroyed for a lack of knowledge, Hosea 4:6.

So, now let me help you incorporate some practical principles to begin to help you reverse Eve's curse and become a healthier you:

-Avoid foods and drinks with high fructose corn syrup and MSG when possible

-Prepare more home-cooked meals; you will be more aware of your food's ingredients

-Plan to eat 4-6 small meals a day to increase and energize your metabolism. If you can prepare your meals or know healthy places to eat at least two days ahead of time, you increase your chances of fueling your body properly. When you eat small meals on a regular basis, you avoid getting hungry. This will prevent you from making bad choices.

-Beware of fad diets and rapid weight loss programs; use the FDA food pyramid as your food guideline

-Drink at least 64 ounces of water every day

to avoid dehydration and hunger

-Take a multi-vitamin to help your body get its proper nutrients

-Eat more organic fruits and vegetables

-Start a stretching program to increase your flexibility; you will feel better

-If possible, exercise in the morning to avoid being sidetracked

-Get at least 8 hours of sleep nightly; this will keep your body rejuvenated

-Find an accountability partner to hold you accountable for achieving your weight loss goals

-Don't procrastinate; start some type of physical activity today

## *Safety First*

Exercising is essential for improving your quality of life. However, safety should be your top priority. Whenever you begin a new exercise regimen, you should design your workout plan to protect joints and strengthen muscle.

Knee and back injuries are the main concerns in health clubs today. People generally put vigorous exercise above safe and proper techniques. The best approach is to learn the proper techniques in order to preserve your body for the long haul. It doesn't make much sense to exercise now and then 20 years down the road, your doctor has to recommend a walker because of the wear and tear on your body.

How many times have you seen "that guy at the gym that can bench press 300 pounds screaming at the top of his lungs using awful form?" How healthy is that? Let's take a moment to learn how to work our bodies from the inside out rather than the outside in. This simply means we should begin our workout plan with light weights to strengthen our joints first. Most people often start a workout plan with heavy weights to receive immediate gratification, instead of working to achieve the long-term benefits. When you start with lighter weights, you have better control and it reduces the possibility of injuries.

I would suggest when doing cardiovascular activities, such as aerobic activity, wearing proper shoes is a must! A top quality aerobic or cross trainer shoe is recommended. Remember to start slow. Work within your own fitness level. Avoid trying to keep up with people that have been training longer than you have. Also remember, before you start any type of fitness program, to consult a physician so that you are aware of your physical capabilities within a workout regimen.

## *Ten Ways to Flatten Your Stomach*

If you're like most people, your stomach is the one part of your body that is a major struggle and it's usually the last thing you get rid of. No amount of abdominal exercises will reveal well-toned muscles if you are padding them with an extra layer of fat. If you're still hanging on to some extra pounds, this is the area where they are probably hidden. Abs are very stubborn; other parts of your body, such as your legs, will reveal your training efforts and muscle tone more quickly because they are less prone to store fat. This is not true with the abdominal area. Drastic change in this area requires hard work. Remember your abdominal area's condition is 80% diet, so you must watch

> Just keep in mind 10-20 well-executed crunches are more beneficial than 50 sloppy ones!

what you eat. Unfortunately, the body is designed to store fat in the abdominal area. That's why it's not easy to achieve a perfectly flat abdomen and in some cases, it's impossible! But you can greatly improve your abdominal area and end up with a nice midsection that suits your body type by just following these tips:

*-In your workout program, each week perform different abdominal exercises. This system is effective in keeping your abdominal muscles constantly challenged, which speeds up results.*

*-When you perform your abdominal routine, put all of your focus on the abdominal area. If don't focus on what you are doing, it is very easy to allow other muscles to do some of the work and your abdominal muscles won't get fatigued or toned.*

*-When working your abs, practice proper breathing techniques; always exhale on the exertion.*

*-Eating habits are just as critical to a lean midsection. Replace sodium, sugar and preservative-laden foods with fresh whole unprocessed foods. Drink as much water as you can all day long to flush away bloating. Consuming ice chilled water will allow you to burn a few extra calories as your body works to warm up. Also keep your diet*

balanced, and eat a healthy ratio of carbohydrates, fats and proteins. And keep in mind, calories do count. Eating too many calories—whether they are fats, carbohydrates or proteins—will keep you padded in the midsection area!

-Avoid carbonated and alcoholic beverages; they have been associated with a rise in cortisol, a stress hormone that produces fat around the midsection.

-To burn a few extra calories, try doing cardiovascular exercise at least three to five times a week. Including a regular cardiovascular exercise routine can help burn some of the extra fat. This will help expose the muscle that you are building.

-If you've lost extra body fat and still don't see well-toned abdominal muscles, increase your repetitions when performing abdominal exercises. If your abs are not fatigued with 25 or 50 repetitions, add another 10 or 20 more. Just keep in mind, 10 or 20 well-executed crunches are more beneficial than 50 sloppy ones!

-Working your abs every other day is a sufficient workout. However, if you would like to be more aggressive, that's great! You won't over-train your abs unless you are adding heavy weights or are extremely sore.

-Finally, train your abdominal muscles by simply keeping them contracted when performing all of your other *exercises; when sitting, standing or driving. Consciously, holding them in can reduce back strain and help to flatten your entire midsection.*

## *Armed and Fabulous*

You may know the back of your upper arm as the part that keeps on waving long after the rest of your arm has stopped. That's because this is an area where many women tend to store excess body fat. While you can't "spot reduce," though aerobic exercise will help by reducing overall body fat, you can tone and tighten this area; thus resulting in smaller, firmer-looking arms.

Most women fear that weight training will bulk them up and take away their feminine nature. This is not true because female testosterone levels are not high enough to cause this to happen. Don't worry; pumping iron is the best way to achieve fabulous arms.

The upper arm consists of two major muscle groups: the triceps and the biceps. The triceps runs along the back of the arm from the shoulder to the elbow; it straightens or extends the arm serving as the pushing muscle (e.g., pushing a baby stroller).

And the biceps runs from the front of the shoulder to the inside of the elbow which flexes the arm to work as the lifting muscle. That's the muscle that helps you pick up that heavy shopping bag at the Macy's Red Dot sale.

Toned and shapely arms are well within your reach. The following exercises will help you reshape your upper arms so they appear leaner and more defined.

*-TRICEP DIPS: Sit on the edge of a chair with your feet on the floor, knees bent with your hands close to your body with your fingers wrapped around the corners of the chair thumbs facing forward. Straighten your arms and lift your buttocks up and in front of the chair seat. Slowly bend your elbows as far as comfortably possible, allowing your hips to drop below the level of the chair seat. Straighten your arms and lift your back to seat level.*

Keep your elbows close to your body; keep your buttocks close to the chairs as you lower. Do not push out and away from the chair; to intensify the exercise, straighten your legs by placing your feet farther from the chair; to simplify bring the feet closer and bend your knees more.

-BICEP CURLS: *Depending on your fitness level, grab an 8-10-pound dumbbell in each hand. Raise the weights one at a time in a controlled motion; lowering is just as important, if not more important, than lifting the weight. You should perform bicep curls on the same days you do your tricep dips, so that you evenly distribute the weight-bearing exercise to your arms. If you can do more than 15 repetitions without a struggle, you may need to increase the size of your weights, which can be purchased at your local Walmart or Target inexpensively.*

## Stability Ball Exercises

### Super Squats with an Exercise Ball

Stand with the exercise ball propped between your lower (lumbar) spine and a wall, pressing slightly into the ball. With hands at your sides or on hips, check that your feet are hip-width apart and slightly in front of you; bending your knees and hips, slowly move into a sitting position with your knees over your ankles. Keep the ball in contact with your back as you move. Return to standing position, keeping the ball in contact with your back as you move.

### *Perform 3 sets of 15 reps*

## Bridges with an Exercise Ball

Sit on the exercise ball with your hands on your hips or crossed on your chest. Walk forward, gradually rolling the ball out until it supports your head and shoulders instead of your buttocks. As you roll out, be sure to keep your weight on top of the ball. Form a flat "tabletop" with your hips, shoulders, and knees aligned—and your feet flat on the floor directly under your knees, without moving the ball, lower and lift your hips, tightening muscles in your buttocks and back of your thighs.

*Perform 3 sets of 15 reps*

## Power Push-Ups with an Exercise Ball

Lie face down with the exercise ball underneath your belly and your palms flat on the floor. Use your hands to walk out to a plank position resting the ball anywhere from your hips to your ankles (this should be a position that provides for a challenging push-up, but allows your spine to stay aligned with ears, shoulders and hips in a line.) Bend your elbows to lower your upper body toward the floor, keeping your shoulders away from your ears and your abdominal muscles engaged.

*Perform 3 sets of 25 reps*

## Abdominal Crunch with an Exercise Ball

Get into a push-up position with the exercise ball under your knees and your palms flat on the floor. Tuck your knees in toward your chest as the ball rolls toward your ankles. Return to the starting position, staying balanced on the ball.

*Perform 3 sets of 50 reps*

## Hamstring and Butt Curls with an Exercise Ball

Lie on your back with the exercise ball under your heels and your palms flat on the floor. Lift hips slightly and bend your knees to draw the ball toward your buttocks, without moving your hips.

*Perform 3 sets of 15 reps*

## Walk-Outs with an Exercise Ball

Rest your belly on the exercise ball with hands and toes on the floor. Walk out your hands to a plank position with the ball under your ankles, then walk back trying to keep the ball under your body.

*Perform 3 sets of 15 reps*

## *Controlling Your Weight with Nutrition*

Let's talk about how to combine the proper micro-nutrients to help fat loss. First of all, micro-nutrients are your protein, carbohydrates and essential fatty acids. When you eat these nutrients in the right combination, they will help you burn fat more rapidly. The start of any successful exercise program is laying a proper nutritional foundation. Trying to start a regimen without the right balance of carbs, fats, vitamins and minerals can be harmful to the body long term.

Carbohydrates provide the body with energy; they are divided in two groups: simple carbs and complex carbs. Simple carbs include sugar, which is found in fruits and candy. Complex carbs are starch-based foods such as pasta and rice. Although carbs are good for the body, too many can be a problem because they break down into sugar, which produces unwanted fat. One way to prevent this is to never eat carbohydrates alone. Always eat your carbs with proteins and essential fatty acids. It is best to eat carbohydrates before a training session for energy, and afterward to replenish. As a general rule, you should aim to get around 60% of your daily caloric intake from carbs.

Protein is the building block for muscle and provides the body with the necessary nutrients to help repair the body after a vigorous workout. Good sources of protein include meats (if you must), fish and nuts. Aim to get about 15% of your calories from proteins by consuming a small amount during every meal.

Fats normally get bad press because most people feel they are unhealthy to eat. Fats are a great source of energy and provide a protective layer around the organs. Saturated fats, such as those found in dairy products and in red meats, are high in cholesterol, which clogs your arteries, leads to high blood pressure and can cause heart disease. On the other hand, mono- and polyunsaturated fats such as those found in oily fish, nuts and wheat germ oil, are much healthier for you.

> Always eat your carbs with proteins and essential fatty acids.

Vitamins and minerals are essential for good health and proper growth. Eating properly will help provide the body with the right vitamins and minerals. In addition, a regular supplementation of vitamins will help your body get the accurate amount of nutrients where foods fall short.

The key is to always plan ahead. To realize the full benefits of living a healthier more energized life, a good plan should consist of the following formula: 60% nutrition, 30% fitness and 10% rest. By following this plan you are on your way to a healthier lifestyle!

It has been my pleasure to take this journey with you. I am glad you have committed to a healthy lifestyle. Remember nutrition is just as important as exercise; you must do both. Let me leave you with this:

REMEMBER ALWAYS LOVE YOURSELF
BELIEVE IN YOURSELF
PUT GOD FIRST IN EVERYTHING YOU SAY AND DO
WATCH WHAT YOU EAT AND DRINK
BE FIT, FINE AND GENUINE—
AND BELIEVE YOU CAN DO IT

# ABOUT THE AUTHOR

Sharon Page is a former Flight Attendant, Co-Author and Writer for *Sister2Sister Magazine*. As a Health and Wellness Consultant for Ardyss International, she has taught thousands of women around the world how to "Create Wealth While Promoting Health." Page is a powerful Coach, Speaker and Trainer with a mission to educate women on the importance of maintaining a healthy lifestyle.

For a schedule of appearances or bookings, visit www.eatyourfoodnaked.com

You may email the Author at eatyourfoodnaked@gmail.com

To order reshaping garments or nutritional products, please visit www.ardysslife.com/sculptyourbody

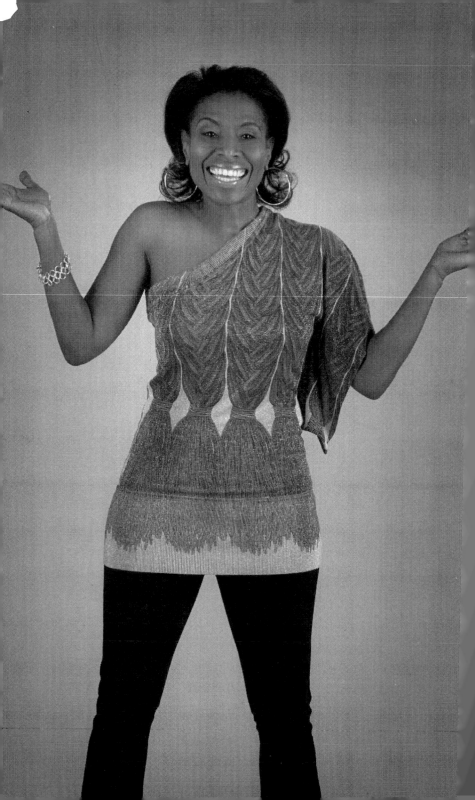